Heal Your Back

T0270646

Heal Your Back

4 steps to a pain-free life

Anisha Joshi

Vermilion
LONDON

Vermilion, an imprint of Ebury Publishing
One Embassy Gardens, 8 Viaduct Gdns,
Nine Elms, London SW11 7BW

Vermilion is part of the Penguin Random House group of companies
whose addresses can be found at global.penguinrandomhouse.com

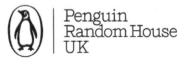

Penguin
Random House
UK

First published by Vermilion in 2024

www.penguin.co.uk

A CIP catalogue record for this book is available from the British Library

ISBN 9781785044670

Typeset in 11/15.25 pt Sabon LT W1G by Jouve (UK), Milton Keynes
Printed and bound in Great Britain by Clays Ltd, Elcograf S.p.A.

Illustrations by Emily Voller

The authorised representative in the EEA is Penguin Random House Ireland,
Morrison Chambers, 32 Nassau Street, Dublin D02 YH68

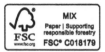

The information in this book has been compiled as general guidance on the specific
subjects addressed. It is not a substitute and not to be relied on for medical advice.
So far as the author is aware the information given is correct and up to date as at
June 2024. Practice, laws and regulations all change and the reader should obtain
up-to-date professional advice on any such issues. The author and publishers disclaim,
as far as the law allows, any liability arising directly or indirectly from the use,
or misuse, of the information contained in this book.

Contents

Introduction

WELCOME TO *Heal Your Back*. Whatever led to you picking up this book, I hope that the information you find here will help you reclaim your happiness, positivity and energy, which may have been drained by your back pain.

There's no doubt that back pain can adversely affect the whole body and people's overall quality of life. Around 84 per cent of adults experience back pain at some point in their lives[1] and, according to public service union UNISON, this contributes to more than 12 million working days lost every year in the UK.[2] Since 2020, there has been a 291 per cent increase in the number of people who are coming into my clinic seeking answers for why they have suddenly started to get back pain. These statistics are exactly why I feel it's necessary to shine a light on back pain wherever I can. The more people talk about it, the more they will realise that it happens all the time to so many of us.

I believe that pain is a signal for change. As an osteopath with three busy clinics, I have worked with thousands of people from all over the world who have suffered from back pain of all kinds. And this book is the result of all of that experience, bringing you the tools and techniques that I know to have proven results with my patients. I have had the honour of treating people who have been completely overwhelmed and fatigued by their ongoing pain, and watching them free

1

themselves from seemingly never-ending daily symptoms. I have witnessed first hand how implementing physical practices, such as building in movement and exercise – something that you love and find fun! – as well as some potentially surprising strategies, such as changing your mindset and making small changes to your diet, all of which we will explore in this book, can help people just like you to heal, grow and flourish beyond their back pain.

The body's ability to heal itself is greater than you realise.

Pain is usually down to many factors and you need to look after all elements of it to truly heal. Addressing both your physical and mental health is key to making changes that last and will enable you to heal in more ways than you imagined.

Many of my clients are lost, confused or anxious about their recovery, but more than anything, it's apparent that their lack of knowledge is the true worry. By giving you the tools and information in this book, I want to change that. Using evidence-based research, I want to help you to understand the real causes of spinal pain (often rooted in the mental and physical stresses and strains of the modern world) and truly empower you to take control of your back, overcome your pain and live a healthier, happier life – pain free.

How to Use This Book

I wrote this book to help you understand your pain and your back in a super simple and concise way. I've therefore split it into three parts and, ideally, I'd like you to read each chapter consecutively. By the end of this book, you'll see that you can find the keys to healing within your own body, with understanding and a few important tweaks to your habits and daily movement patterns.

The thing about pain and discomfort is that if we don't understand the causes, then it seems much scarier and debilitating than it actually is. A good example of this is if you blindfold someone and then ask them to put their hand into a box to identify an unknown object; it is highly likely that they will be nervous and will think it might hurt them. However, if you show them what it is that they are touching, they don't feel as nervous – and that is what this book is about. It is about taking off your blindfold to pain and hopefully giving you the tools to better manage yours.

Before we get stuck into the nitty-gritty of how to heal your back with the four steps (starting on page 71), it's therefore important we do a deep dive into the anatomy of bones, ligaments and muscles (hello to the anatomy geeks out there!). In Part 1, we'll delve into the detail of exactly how the spine works, to understand the nuts and bolts of this incredible mechanism inside us, which houses and protects the core of our nervous system, is the fulcrum of our balance and influences so much of our strength and daily abilities. We'll also look at how we absolutely can optimise our back health and prevent some of the most common back pain issues, as long as we know how.

If you're not too fussed about learning about the anatomy and just want to know how to stop your pain, don't worry, I've got your back (pun intended) – I promise you will find it as fascinating as I do, as you will see how incredible and magical your body truly is! In order to learn how to manage and prevent your back pain, it is crucial that you understand how your back – and specifically pain – can be influenced by other physical – and often emotional – systems.

We'll also look at the different types of back pain, as well as the causes and symptoms. This understanding will benefit you when moving into the more practical steps in Part 2 for helping yourself out of your back pain.

When I first see clients in clinic, I request a full medical case history, taking their entire lifestyle into consideration, including their activity levels, stress levels, nutrition and sleep – all of which can impact pain. In the same way, in Part 2, I'll show you how you can access and nurture the wonderful systems within you to be able to live a life free from back pain using a simple four-step approach:

1. Keep moving: Keeping our bodies in motion is crucial for a healthy back. We need to get off our duffs and wiggle those buns. Regular exercise and stretching can help strengthen our back muscles, improve flexibility, increase blood flow to the area and reduce pain.

2. Reset your mind: Our minds are powerful things. Maintaining a positive attitude and keeping stress at bay can do wonders for your back pain.

3. Eat well: Opting for a balanced diet rich in fruits, veggies, lean proteins and wholegrains helps reduce any inflammation in the body, which, as you'll discover, has a positive effect on pain. It also helps to maintain a healthy weight, reducing the strain on your back and giving you more energy to tackle the day.

4. Sleep better: Good-quality sleep isn't just about counting sheep; it's about finding ways to support a restful night's sleep so you can break the sleep–pain cycle and reduce your back pain.

Part 3 is dedicated to the future and will outline the treatment options available to you, as well as how to overcome any hurdles so you can build these key pillars into your life in the long term. We'll also look at the importance of consistency and managing any pain flare-ups. I always say to my clients that, when it comes to back pain, you need to go towards what you want and not away from what you don't want. Each of the chapters in this book will support you in doing just that.

I want you to see this book as your go-to bible full of practical tips for healing your back. I'm excited to give you the ability to rid yourself of back pain – for life!

WHAT IS OSTEOPATHY?

Osteopathy is a bespoke treatment that utilises medical and musculoskeletal knowledge to help diagnose and treat pain and injury. Osteopaths undergo intensive training over four years, are skilled in diagnostic techniques and work alongside consultants, doctors and other healthcare professionals to ensure the highest level of care.

Osteopathy combines massage techniques, manipulation and exercise rehabilitation, which is an important part of osteopathic care. As we'll cover in Chapter 3, exercises are important to keep the body moving, reduce inflammation and prevent further injury.

Drawing on my extensive experience as an osteopath, I've included tips and exercises throughout the book that you can do at home, as well as anecdotes and case studies to help you understand the impact the four steps, discussed in Part 2, can have in real life, and hopefully make you realise you're not alone in your back pain journey. I have helped thousands of people – from dancers and athletes, to desk workers and manual workers – to feel better about their back, and now it's your turn. I want you to think of me as your little osteopath angel on your shoulder, reminding you every day to think about your back and remember that you do have the power to help yourself heal.

Jump right in with incorporating the practical and mindset tips in this book. Actually commit to doing the exercises you find dotted throughout these pages – ideally implementing at least one tool a week from each step, and more regularly if you can, so that, by the end of the book, you'll have built up a network of new and effective ways to readjust your relationship with pain and heal your back.

In each of the steps in Part 2, I've provided a 'progress tracker' so you can take just 20 seconds to check in with yourself and how you're feeling about your back pain and the various tools I'll be providing you with. This is a great way to realise how far you have come as, initially, the changes you make will be small and, unless you check in like this, you may not even realise that positive changes are happening.

This book is intended to be your resource kit to help you navigate your mindset and emotional response to your back pain, begin to heal it completely and prevent it from recurring, and ultimately make sure your spine is in tip-top health throughout the rest of your life. I'd love you to really use these pages as if you were having a regular one-to-one session with me: highlight your favourite bits in the margins, fold down the pages if you need to, maybe even carry it with you and have it at work as a daily prompt to move more regularly. Consider this book as embodying your new understanding and appreciation of your spine and its incredible ability to heal.

Make this pledge to yourself to regularly return to the information in the book, tracking your pain and mobility in a journal for at least eight weeks, so that you can begin to notice positive shifts. This will ensure that you get the most out of the book and will help you integrate the tools into your daily life. While pain is very individual and you'll all be at different stages of your healing journey, for those of you who would prefer a more structured 'plan', each step includes an eight-week guide outlining gradual steps to implement small changes each week (see pages 112, 146, 184 and 220).

Think of this book as just the beginning of a long-term commitment to listening to and understanding your body and the messages that your aches and discomfort may be giving you, and committing to a life without the pain that is getting you down.

Knowledge Is Power

There is a lot of information in these pages, and some of the anatomy detail may feel complex at first. However, please bear with me, as getting your head around the anatomy will really help you to truly understand the fundamentals that underlie your back pain. So, take some time to reread these sections and familiarise yourself with the language so that you can apply it to your own experience and health more effectively.

While you don't have to be able to remember all of the detail in order for this knowledge to be powerful, you do need to act on it. Knowledge *is* power, but action is more powerful when it comes to back health and preventing and healing your pain. What I will show you in this book is that pain can be complicated, but it can also be simplified. We know that many things contribute to us feeling pain and it's about understanding those things and facing them head on. From my experience as an osteopath over the past 15 years, I know that pain is heavily connected to the emotions that we are feeling – so it's not as simple as approaching a problem solely from a structural or physical angle. I believe and have seen through my practice that pain isn't ever something we have to 'put up with' or 'get used to'. It really is something we can manage and improve, regardless of our age. It is *never* too late.

By picking up this book, you have taken the first step on your healing journey, embracing the fact that you *can* heal your back pain, committing to understanding your body and learning how to implement small but powerful lifestyle changes to improve your back health, for life. It's important to remember that there is no quick fix when it comes to back pain. Instead, the four steps are about developing better habits, for life. Commit to actioning each of the steps for at least eight weeks and think of this book as your road map to a more comfortable, pain-free life, where you have the tools to empower yourself.

This is the beginning of your journey to heal your back – I am with you every step of the way. Let's get started!

PART 1

Understanding Your Back

My aim in this first part of the book is for you to get a greater understanding of the structure of the spine and all the muscles, ligaments and nerves that feed into it, as well as the different types and causes of back pain. There is a lot of information in these pages, and some of the detail may feel complex at first, so I know you'll be tempted to skip it. However, please bear with me, as getting your head around these sections means that you'll be able to apply it to your own experience and health more effectively and understand the remedies to overcome your pain. As I have seen with so many of my clients, with this knowledge, I know you will feel empowered to heal your back and get on board with the four steps in Part 2.

CHAPTER 1

How the Back Works

REMEMBER, KNOWLEDGE IS power. By understanding the crucial role that your back plays in your whole body's strength, balance and function, you can better understand the reasons behind occasional discomfort or even severe back pain, making you less fearful of the pain you're experiencing. My aim is to give you the superpower of knowledge so that you don't panic when you experience a back problem.

Let's kick off with an overview of the spine, looking at the vertebrae, nerves, joints, muscles and ligaments and how, when they are not functioning correctly or are damaged, it can lead to pain.

The Basic Anatomy of the Spine

Many people think of the back as only the lower part, but it actually covers the area from the base of your skull all the way down to where your spine meets your pelvis. The back also contains some of the biggest and strongest muscles in your whole body.

Your spine acts as a fulcrum for most movements in your everyday life – bending down (flexion), arching your back (extension), leaning to one side (lateral flexion), turning your head to look over your shoulder (rotation) or swinging a golf club, playing tennis or lifting and putting your child into a cot/buggy (axial rotation – where the entire body moves around the spine's central axis).

As an osteopath, I see the back as this beautiful, incredibly strong support system that holds us upright and enables our body to help us live our lives, doing the things that we love. Whether it is lifting our children out of their cot, cycling for miles every weekend, running a marathon or giving birth, the back is involved.

Your spine is made up of four areas:

1. Cervical (your neck): has a slight inwards curve called a lordosis.
2. Thoracic (mid-back): has an outwards curve called a kyphosis.
3. Lumbar (lower back): inwards curve.
4. Sacral (lower back): inwards curve.

It is these curves that allow for ultimate movement, performance and strength when going about our day-to-day lives. They work as a seamless team to help keep us upright and moving.

Our spines are all unique to us and if their natural curve is impacted for any reason, it may affect the way in which our muscles attach to the spine and the joints around it, and therefore the amount of pressure that goes through the spine, which can predispose us to muscle pain or even early-onset disc degeneration (see page 19). Things such as moving or lifting heavy objects incorrectly or carrying or lifting something too heavy (for example, carrying four bags of heavy shopping home instead of making multiple trips) can also

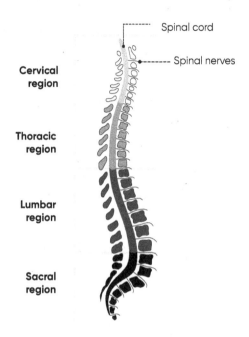

Spinal cord

Spinal nerves

Cervical region

Thoracic region

Lumbar region

Sacral region

contribute to back pain (see page 53 for guidance on a proper lifting technique).

THE SPINAL CORD

The spinal cord runs down the inside of the spine, acting as a communication highway between the brain and the rest of the body, sending messages for movement and sensation. When the spinal cord is damaged, which is a rare occurrence and usually due to trauma like a road traffic accident, it can lead to problems such as difficulty moving or a lack of function in some of your organs – for example, a lack of control over your bowel or bladder. These symptoms are a medical emergency and should be dealt with by specialist doctors.

Each of the four areas of the back has different shaped vertebrae (the bones of the spine itself), so let's continue by exploring those.

Vertebrae

The structure and function of the vertebrae play a pivotal role in our musculoskeletal system, with the spine acting as a central support system for the entire body.

Many of my clients come to me after years of back pain, worrying that their back is going to 'snap' or 'break' from simple things such as bending over to hug a child or unload the dishwasher, for example. But it's so reassuring to know that the 33 individual vertebrae, from the cervical to the lumbar region, contribute to the spine's resilience and ability to bear the body's weight.

I appreciate that for those of you who have ongoing pain, you might be unable to fathom this concept, but in general, your body is the most innovative, powerful machine you will come across. The human body is strong and our vertebrae are perfectly formed to support us and enable us to function as we need to. Your body wants to move, it wants to lift things and it wants to ensure you live life to the fullest. All you need to do is be consistent with looking after it. The spine can bend, resist compression and is highly resistant to fractures. This robustness allows it to resist forces and heal rapidly when subjected to stress or pressure.

The amazing thing about bones is the way in which they grow and increase in density. Bone tissue is constantly being remodelled and repaired, which helps to maintain its strength and integrity over time. As we'll explore in Chapter 3, weight-bearing activities like walking, running and strength training (when you lift weights in order to strengthen the muscles and joints) are good for our bones because they encourage more bone to be laid down. It's a bit like putting loads of people and luggage into your car and the tyres inflating automatically to the optimum level.

However, there are some conditions that can impact bone health:

- Hormones: Hormonal imbalances, such as low or high levels of oestrogen or testosterone – as in thyroid dysfunction, for example – can lead to decreased bone density and increased risk of fractures.
- Medications: Some medications, such as steroids, can weaken bones and increase the risk of fractures. If you are taking medications that may impact your bone health, talk to your doctor about ways to mitigate the effects.
- Age: As people age, their bones naturally become less dense and more fragile, which can increase the risk of fractures.
- Genetics: A family history of osteoporosis (see below) or other bone diseases can increase the risk of developing similar conditions.
- Lifestyle factors: Smoking, excessive alcohol consumption and a sedentary lifestyle can all contribute to poor bone health.

Whether through reduced density, increased fragility or a heightened risk of fractures, these factors show the relationship between skeletal health and pain, particularly in the context of back pain. As we'll come to see, when your bones aren't strong, it can lead to inflammation in your body, which can lead to pain.

OSTEOPOROSIS

Osteoporosis is a condition where your bones become weak and fragile, like a sponge that's lost some of its density. It's kind of like having a house with walls that are easy to break because they're not as strong as they should be. This can make your bones more susceptible to fractures, even from minor bumps or falls. This is why weight-bearing activities like walking, jogging and lifting weights are recommended for this condition to increase the strength of the bones. There is evidence to show that brief bouts of daily weight-bearing exercise can increase your bone density. For example, gently hopping for a few minutes a day can increase the bone density of your hip (femoral head).[1] (See Chapter 3 for more on strength-training exercises.)

My mum has osteoporosis and for a long time she was really worried about it – when you're told by your doctor that you have 'weak' bones, it's easy to panic and not want to do anything. In fact, she would have sat on the sofa wrapped in bubble wrap if she could! However, when I spoke to her about exercise and what it does to your bones, she realised that being scared was the worst thing she could do. She wanted to make that change to her health and so she joined the gym and now swims, walks, strength trains and goes to spin classes. She actually puts me to shame, to be honest, and she is 70!

Other conditions that may affect the vertebrae and lead to pain include but are not limited to:

- Osteophytes (bone spurs): As we get older, small bones a bit like stalagmites can develop on our spinal vertebrae. Sometimes these can grow to be quite large and impinge on nerves, causing pain.
- Spondylolisthesis: This is where one of the vertebrae shifts forwards onto the one below. This can cause lower back pain symptoms.
- Ankylosing spondylitis (AS): This is a long-term condition in which the spine and other areas of the body become inflamed. 'Bamboo spine', which is where the bones in the spine become fused together, is a potential complication of AS that can lead to pain and fractures (though this is rare because, as we've seen, the spine is strong).

Intervertebral discs

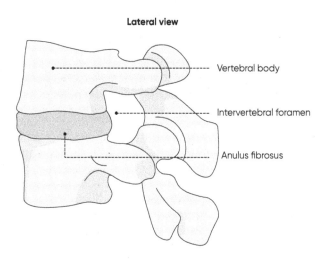

Lateral view

Vertebral body

Intervertebral foramen

Anulus fibrosus

Intervertebral discs are positioned between our vertebrae. They consist of the anulus fibrosus, an outer layer with collagen fibre rings providing strength, and the nucleus pulposus, a gel-like centre that acts as a shock absorber by distributing pressure evenly. Often people compare our discs to a tyre-like structure.

These discs play a vital role in spinal function:

Superior view

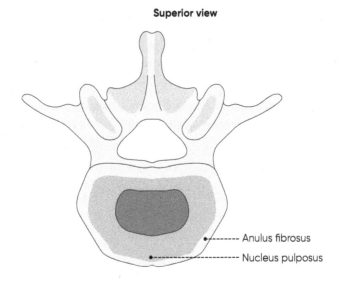

------- Anulus fibrosus

---------- Nucleus pulposus

1. Shock absorption: The nucleus pulposus absorbs and dissipates mechanical forces, preventing excessive impact on the spine during various activities.
2. Flexibility: The layered structure of the anulus fibrosus allows the spine to flex, extend and rotate while maintaining stability.
3. Load distribution: Intervertebral discs distribute the weight of the upper body across the vertebral column, preventing excessive pressure on individual vertebrae.
4. Maintaining spinal height: The water content in the nucleus pulposus contributes to the overall height of the disc and, consequently, the spine.

5. Nutrient exchange: Cartilaginous endplates enable the exchange of nutrients and waste products between the disc and surrounding blood vessels in the vertebral bodies.
6. Support for movement: Intervertebral discs enable smooth movement and articulation between adjacent vertebrae, allowing for a wide range of motion in the spine.

Occasionally, as with the vertebrae themselves, the intervertebral discs can be affected by injury or age. Over time, the water content in the nucleus pulposus tends to decrease, causing the discs to lose some of their height and flexibility. This process is known as 'disc degeneration' and is a natural part of the ageing process. As discs flatten and lose their ability to absorb shock effectively, the risk of conditions such as osteoarthritis – and therefore pain – increases.

Discs can also be subject to injuries and strains, often resulting from activities that involve repetitive or excessive loading of the spine, like competitive lifting. This heavy lifting and sudden, forceful movements can lead to injuries such as disc herniation or prolapse. These conditions can cause the anulus fibrosus to weaken or rupture, allowing the nucleus pulposus to protrude beyond its normal boundaries.

Although the above sounds quite frightening, these injuries are uncommon.

MYTH-BUSTER: 'SLIPPED' DISCS

I hate this term. It's one that was possibly created by the medical profession to help describe a disc injury to patients. Now, I am all for easy explanations of a condition or injury. However, implying that a disc is weak and like a bar of soap that can just slip out of your hands implies that it can happen extremely easily and, once it happens, it's gone – the soap is forever in the bathtub with no means of retrieving it, which just isn't the case.

The truth is that, as we've seen, the structure of a disc is more like a tyre . . . a really expensive one. It has multiple layers and is super strong. It doesn't 'slip'; it prolapses or herniates, which means that sometimes some of the interior material of the disc comes out. Disc protrusions or herniations most commonly occur in 20–50-year-olds, though they only account for about 4 per cent of back pain cases.[2,3,4]

The most interesting thing about this is that studies have shown that not every disc injury leads to pain and it impacts people in different ways. Broken bones always have a pain response, but discs do not, and the theory behind this is that our bodies adapt to a slow change. In one study, researchers performed magnetic resonance imaging (MRI) scans on the backs of 311 people who had no history of back pain or sciatica (pain going down the leg from the lower back). The MRI scans showed that 37 per cent of the participants had at least one disc bulge and 30 per cent had at least one disc protrusion. However, only 1.3 per cent of the participants reported experiencing back pain or sciatica during the 12 months following the MRI scans.[5] It is important to note, however, that not all disc prolapses will be asymptomatic.

If the disc protrusion is sudden, it can cause excruciating pain and, if it is touching the nerve, there will be even more discomfort as it may lead to sciatica. Sudden disc protrusions can occur as part of the natural ageing process when the disc dehydrates and weakens the nucleus pulposus. In younger people this can happen as a result of trauma, like falling over or bending over very quickly to pick up a heavy child.

For others, if the disc prolapse is gradual over time, the structures around it are able to adapt, and so those with disc injuries may experience no pain whatsoever and can keep living their life unaffected. Additionally, while there are many who do require a surgery called a discectomy to reduce their symptoms, there is also research to show that half of disc herniations spontaneously get better and deherniate (meaning they go back to where they need to be).[6]

Nerves

Nerves are specialised cells that transmit information throughout the body. The nerve supply to the *entire* body comes from your spine, and there are a *lot* of nerves in your body – over 7 trillion in fact.

Nerves can be split into three main types:

1. Sensory nerves: These nerves carry information from the body's sensory organs, such as the eyes, ears, nose and skin, to the brain. They allow us to see, hear, smell, taste and feel sensations such as touch, pressure and temperature.
2. Motor nerves: When the brain sends a signal to a motor nerve, it triggers a series of events that cause the muscle to contract and produce movement. Without motor

nerves, our muscles would be unable to receive the signals they need to move.

3. Autonomic nerves: These nerves control the involuntary functions of the body, such as breathing, heart rate and digestion.

Sometimes nerves can malfunction. They can over-fire, be hypersensitive or under-reactive – all of which can lead to pain, weakness or instability within the body. Infections like shingles can cause nerve pain, as can conditions such as multiple sclerosis, carpal tunnel syndrome, diabetes (in the form of diabetic neuropathy) and stroke. However, these conditions are all quite rare and the main nerve pain I see in my clinic is trapped nerves.

In terms of back pain, nerves are critical. Nociceptors, which are specialised nerve cells that detect pain, are located throughout the body and start at your spine. When these cells are activated by tissue damage or inflammation, they send signals to the brain that are interpreted as pain. This allows us to recognise when something is wrong and take appropriate action to protect ourselves. We'll further explore this when we look at the different types of pain in the next chapter (see page 39).

Nerves and their intricate network of signalling pathways are essential for the experience of pain. They not only convey information about potential threats to our body, but also contribute to the way we perceive and respond to pain.

The transmission of pain signals involves several steps:

1. Detection: Nociceptors detect harmful stimuli at the site of injury or irritation.

2. Transmission: Once activated, nociceptors generate electrical signals, which are then transmitted along nerve fibres, specifically the A-delta and C fibres. A-delta fibres transmit sharp, immediate pain sensations, while C fibres convey dull, throbbing or burning pain.

3. Spinal cord: The pain signals travel to the spinal cord, where they are relayed to different layers of neurons. In the spinal cord, the signals can be modulated or amplified based on the context and intensity of the pain.

4. Brain interpretation: The spinal cord then transmits the signals to various regions of the brain, including the thalamus and cerebral cortex, which are responsible for processing sensory information and interpreting pain. The brain assigns meaning to the pain sensation, determining its location, intensity and emotional context.

5. Perception: The brain interprets the incoming signals and generates the conscious perception of pain. This perception of pain is influenced by various factors, including personal experiences, emotions, cognitive processes and cultural background.

When you injure yourself, the nerves send signals to your brain that cause the release of the pain chemical, and this can mean your body can heal the area by sending inflammation there.

WHAT IS INFLAMMATION?

Inflammation is the body's natural way of protecting an area and also healing it. When something is wrong, such as tissue damage, your body sends more blood to the

---

area, which can make it red and warm. This blood flows to the cells to help repair and heal. Once the problem is fixed, your body stops the inflammation and things get better. But too much inflammation for a long time can cause issues, so your body has to balance it carefully. Inflammation is a natural response of the body to injury or infection, but chronic inflammation can contribute to various health problems, including pain.

When inflammation is constant in your body, it can also send signals to your brain that make it remember the initial injury. For example, a whiplash injury after a car accident may result in neck pain. If your body experiences stress or sleeps awkwardly, which results in some neck soreness, this inflammation may take your brain back to the traumatic event of having a car accident. It is this inflammation or stiffness that turns into a stress-provoking reaction or catastrophising, which we'll further explore in Chapter 4.

Inflammation is both positive and negative for the body – it enables our bodies to heal the area, but sometimes it can also cause a limitation in movement.

Joints

Joints are where two bones connect. I like to split the joints in our bodies into three categories:

1. Non-moving joints: An example of this is our skull (cranial bones), once the cranial bones have 'ossified' (fused together) and become one plate after birth. They can also be described as fibrous joints. Another example

is our teeth, which are joined to our jaws by a ligament called the periodontal ligament, a fibrous tissue that holds our teeth in their sockets.

2. Slightly moveable joints: These can be further split, but we have a few fibrous joints that are held together with interosseous membranes. A good example of this would be the ribcage and how it moves to enable us to breathe, but also protects our vital organs underneath. There are also slightly moveable cartilaginous joints, which are joints that have cartilage between them. Our pubic symphysis, which is at the front of our pelvis where it fuses between our legs, is a slightly moveable joint that is commonly impacted in pregnancy with a condition called symphysis pubis dysfunction (SPD – see box below). There are also our sacroiliac joints, which are at the back of our pelvis, at the base of our spine. Some people have dimples in their back where these two joints are located.

3. Freely moving joints: These are the main functional parts of our skeleton and body. Articular cartilage covers the surface of each bone and between these is synovial fluid, which is a concoction of filtered blood plasma that looks like egg white. Then you have the outer articular capsule, which is like the strong tendons and ligaments that keep it moving and all together. Freely moving joints also have six subsections:

    a. ball and socket joint: for example, the shoulder or hip
    b. hinge joint: for example, the elbow, knee or wrist
    c. planar joint: for example, the collarbone and spinal vertebrae
    d. saddle joint: where your hand bones meet your fingers

e. pivot joint: the top of your neck
f. condyloid joint: the tiny joints at the base of your fingers

When all of these joints fulfil their purpose and our bodies are functioning correctly and efficiently, this can help to prevent back pain.

Spinal joints are what enable us to move. Some of the key joints in our back are:

1. Vertebral joints: These are the joints between individual vertebrae in the spine. There are several types of vertebral joints, including:
    *   Intervertebral discs (see page 17).
    *   Facet joints: There are two synovial facet joints between each individual spinal segment. For example, there are five lower (lumbar) vertebrae and there are ten facet joints. Facet joints guide and restrict movement of the spine, helping with stability and flexibility.
2. Sacroiliac joints: These are the joints between the sacrum (the triangular bone at the base of the spine) and the iliac bones of the pelvis. They support the weight of the upper body and manage weight bearing from your spine and into your legs.
3. Costovertebral joints: These are the joints between the ribs and the thoracic vertebrae. They provide stability to the ribcage and also allow some degree of movement during breathing.
4. Costotransverse joints: These are the joints between the ribs and the side of your mid-back (thoracic)

vertebrae. They assist in breathing and contribute to overall spine stability.

5. Atlanto-occipital joint: This is the joint between the atlas (first cervical vertebra, C1) and the occipital bone at the base of the skull. It allows for nodding movements of the head.

6. Atlantoaxial joint: This is the joint between the atlas and the axis (second cervical vertebra, C2). It allows for rotation of the head.

7. Lumbosacral joint: This is the joint between the fifth lumbar vertebra (L5) and the sacrum. It plays a role in supporting the body when you're putting load onto the joints, such as when running or lifting things.

SYMPHYSIS PUBIS DYSFUNCTION (SPD)

SPD is a condition affecting the joint at the front of the pelvis connecting the pubic bones. It is most common during pregnancy due to increased ligament flexibility caused by hormonal changes. SPD leads to pain in the pelvic region, lower back, thighs and perineal area. Patients who come into clinic with this also report a sense of instability and difficulty in activities like walking or climbing stairs. The condition is characterised by joint misalignment and instability, often exacerbated by hormonal changes. Treatment includes manual techniques, soft tissue manipulation and exercises to strengthen the pelvic muscles. The main thing is to focus on promoting stability and managing pain, as it can be quite debilitating. Chapters 3 and 5 provide some tips on keeping moving, as well as looking at your nutrition and implementing an anti-inflammatory diet, both of which can help with SPD pain.

SACROILIAC JOINT PAIN

Sacroiliac pain, which is often identified as lower back pain, affects the joint connecting the sacrum and the ilium in the pelvis. This discomfort can stem from various factors such as injury, repetitive stress and pregnancy. The pain typically radiates from the lower back down to the buttocks and sometimes into the thighs. Patients often describe a feeling of 'weakness' in the lower back and hips, which can impact daily activities like walking or bending forwards.

Treatment mainly involves a combination of manual therapy, targeted exercises to strengthen the lower back and core pelvic muscles, and techniques to promote joint stability. Managing pain and enhancing stability are primary goals in addressing sacroiliac pain, as it can significantly impact mobility and quality of life.

Quite often, as our spine acts a bit like scaffolding for our body in terms of holding us up, if other joints in our body aren't functioning efficiently, our back can compensate for it and predispose us to back pain. For example, if you injure your knee falling over, then you may limp while it is sore. It is this act of limping and your body trying to bear weight on the opposite side that can lead to pain in the back where the muscles are working harder than they are used to. Joint pain can also be due to an instability within the joint, arthritis within the joint or referred pain from another part of the body.

The term 'wear and tear' is often used to describe what is happening to someone's spine if they have symptoms that point to osteoarthritis in their spine or joints. I'm not a fan of this term as it gives the impression that your joints are wearing and tearing, and it can mean that patients adapt their activities out of fear that they'll do more damage or cause more pain.

The truth is that osteoarthritis is a normal part of the ageing process and 'wear and tear' is a term used to describe this in a non-medical way. However, I try to reframe this with my clients and remind them that this isn't what is actually happening to their joints. I refer to it as 'normal wear' so they can shift their mindset. What machine doesn't need bits replacing or parts oiling the older it gets? For example, if a bike is not tended to, the chain will get creaky and will snap. Our bodies need the same upkeep and loving attention, and respond to regular maintenance. This *does not* mean that all of us will experience pain, though. Most of the time our body adapts to these gradual changes. Your life isn't over, and having normal wear or osteoarthritis is no reason to give up on activities you enjoy – trust me.

MYTH-BUSTER: 'YOUR BACK IS OUT OF ALIGNMENT'

I spent four years at university being told that structural differences in our bodies were one of the causes of pain. This includes things like spinal curvatures, leg length discrepancies and tilted pelvises. Since the early 2000s there have been many research studies that have shown that these differences *do not* in fact cause back pain.[7,8] As an osteopath, I feel that these slight differences may

---

impact the way in which you move, and consequently this can lead to discomfort and muscle imbalances causing referred pain, as explained above.

Muscles

Muscle issues are probably the most common cause of back pain that I see in my clinic. Muscles are like the engines that help your body move. They're made of tiny muscle cells that can shrink and stretch. These cells have special proteins that pull and push, making the muscles contract. Blood vessels bring them food and oxygen, while connective tissues hold everything in place. Nerves act like remote controls, telling the muscles when to start and stop. So, muscles are a mix of cells, proteins, blood tubes, strong strings and nerve switches that work together to let you move around! The two main muscle groups around your spine are called flexors and extensors, and they are based on either side of your spine. Not only do they support your spine, but ultimately these muscles help with everyday movements.

The body is a beautiful thing and it's also incredibly complicated because it's so interconnected. At the top of the back, your head attaches to your cervical spine and all your neck and shoulder muscles. At the base of your spine, your pelvis and sacrum have your hamstrings, quads and glutes attached to them. Many of the muscles that attach to our spine also attach to various joints throughout the spine and upper body, enabling them to work together to provide stability, movement and support to the back and surrounding areas. An example of this is how our trapezius muscle in our back also attaches to both our shoulders, and how our psoas muscle attaches to our hip. All the muscles in our back – from the neck to the lower back and pelvis – interlink, overlap and connect to one another. Consequently, it's very common for someone to visit my clinic with pain in their neck that then develops into lower back pain. This is because the muscles and nerve supply all overlap so much that tightness and pain in one muscle can lead to tightness and pain in another.

Often my clients think they have 'torn' a muscle, but a 'tear' is incredibly rare in your lower back. It is much more likely that you have *strained* a muscle. A strain is often also described as a 'pulled muscle', which is when the muscle is stretched too far and results in pain.

When you lift weights, your muscles undergo a process called 'muscle hypertrophy'. This process involves the muscle fibres breaking down and causing microtears, and then repairing themselves, resulting in an increase in muscle size and strength over time. With consistent strength training and proper nutrition, your muscles adapt and become stronger to handle heavier weights. How amazing is that? Don't forget how phenomenal and strong our bodies are; even if you have recurrent pain, there's always a way to make your back stronger.

WHAT HAPPENS WHEN YOU STRAIN, SPRAIN OR PULL A MUSCLE?

1. Microscopic damage: When you suddenly push a muscle beyond its usual limits, the muscle fibres

---

can get overstretched. This creates tiny injuries in the muscle tissue.

2. Inflammation: As a response to the damage, your body's immune system starts to send white blood cells and other healing substances to the injured area. This leads to inflammation.

3. Pain and discomfort: The inflammation and damage can cause pain, swelling and discomfort in the area of the strained muscle. You might feel pain when you move the muscle or even when you're resting.

4. Muscle spasm: The body's natural reaction to injury is to protect the area. Muscles around the strained area might tense up or spasm to try to limit movement and protect the injured muscle.

LIGAMENTS AND TENDONS

Ligaments and tendons are both types of connective tissue in the body, but they have different functions and structures. Ligaments connect bones to other bones and provide stability to joints, and they are made up of tough, fibrous tissue that is designed to withstand tension and stretching forces and hold our spinal vertebrae securely in place. Tendons, on the other hand, connect muscles to bones and allow for movement. They are also made up of fibrous tissue, but they are more elastic than ligaments.

A ligament or tendon injury in the spine may manifest as whiplash or an injury like overarching your back on a trampoline and landing awkwardly. Usually this feels similar to an acute muscle spasm and can also radiate across the back. Injuries such as this vary in degrees of pain.

Unlike muscles, which receive a significant blood supply, ligaments and tendons have a relatively poor blood supply, which means they may take longer to heal after an injury because they receive fewer nutrients and oxygen from the blood. Additionally, ligaments and tendons are under constant stress and tension as they need to hold bones and muscles together while allowing for controlled and safe movement, which can also slow down the healing process. When a ligament or tendon is injured, it may take longer to heal because the fibres are constantly being stretched and pulled while we move in everyday life, making it difficult for new tissue to form.

The severity of a ligament or tendon injury can also impact the healing process. Minor sprains or strains may heal within a few weeks, while more severe injuries like a complete tear of a ligament or tendon may require surgery and a longer recovery time.

FASCIA

Fascia is connective tissue that surrounds muscles, bones, nerves and organs throughout the body. It is made of collagen and other proteins, and its function is to provide support and protection to the body's structures while also allowing for movement. If the fascia becomes restricted through lack of movement and potentially dehydration, it can contribute to back pain by limiting the range of movement in the muscles and joints.

How Important Is Posture?

I will be honest and say that I was taught at university that bad posture gives you a bad back, or a hunchback. However, we now know that 'bad posture' doesn't necessarily contribute to the shape of your spine changing. When I tell someone this, they are shocked, as they have heard it their entire life! They look like I've just told them that their hair will fall out if they eat sugar.

'Good posture' is not as important as you think when it comes to back pain.

'Bad' posture is often described as rounded shoulders, head down and slumping forwards when standing or sitting.

When you slump like this, your chest caves in, reducing the space for your diaphragm to function optimally. The diaphragm is a large, dome-shaped muscle that plays a crucial role in the process of breathing. It is located just below the ribcage, separating the chest cavity (thoracic cavity) from the abdominal cavity. The diaphragm is the primary muscle responsible for inhaling and exhaling, and it contracts and relaxes to create changes in lung volume, allowing us to breathe. This compression can limit the diaphragm's ability to contract fully during inhalation, causing your breathing to become shallow. Shallow breathing can impact the function of your diaphragm and the diaphragm attaches to your lumbar spine (the lower back), therefore predisposing you to lower back pain.

However, while the position we hold our bodies in (aka our posture) can compromise their function, 'bad' posture is not the only culprit that can predispose you to back pain and discomfort. Traditional understanding of 'good posture' may be flawed as well – we are taught that 'good posture' is holding yourself rigidly upright, 'shoulders back and down', as if balancing a book on your head. Whether it's desk work, factory work or anything that involves sitting or standing in the same position for a while, being held in a fixed, tense position is going to contribute to the pain someone is experiencing. So this means that, even if you sit in a chair with your back straight like a royal princess or prince for a long period of time, you will *still* get back pain. It's important to understand that it's the positions that are static and held for long periods that are the issue here. *Moving more* is what your spine needs to function healthily. (See Chapter 3 for more on how regular movement is key to relieving back pain, as well as page 44 for my seated desk mobility routine.) Truly 'good' posture is a balanced position that minimises strain on the muscles and spine.

Being aware of your posture and your positioning is essential intel here, to bring some conscious understanding of the way you hold yourself during the day: at your desk, when you're standing waiting for the bus, when you're sitting on the sofa, even where your eyes tend to focus *most of the time*. Therefore, reframing what 'posture' means is important. Good posture isn't 'sitting up straight' in a rigid way, it is ensuring your body is in the best possible alignment and muscle balance, and being consciously aware of your postural habits more of the time. There is a saying that 'the best posture is your next posture', which means that shifting your position throughout the day and becoming more mindful of how you are positioned through practices like yoga, Pilates and meditation can benefit you (see pages 94 and 126 for more on this) and make it less likely that you will experience postural pain.

Posture correctors

I'm not a big fan of posture correctors: adjustable back braces that you wear. My reasons for this are varied, but the main one is that they encourage the belief that 'poor posture is bad for you'. Instead of relying on posture correctors, the following two exercises are a great way to bring your shoulders back by strengthening the correct muscles:

- Rhomboids: Interlace your fingers behind your back and draw your shoulders down and back. Hold this for ten seconds. Repeat 5–6 times, 2–3 times a day.
- Serratus anterior: Place your hands on a wall in front of you (as if you were about to do a standing press-up), squeeze your shoulder blades together and hold for ten seconds. Repeat 10–15 times, once a day.

See page 242 for more on back braces.

OSTEO TOP TIP

If you find yourself often slumping in your chair and you have lower back pain, take a deep breath into your tummy, without moving your position. Exhale and then move your position slightly – bring your shoulders back, sit up straight and take another deep breath. Do you feel the difference in how much more healthy oxygen your lungs can take in and how much pain you are experiencing?

As complicated as our back is, it is likely the most innovative machine you'll ever see. Our back, muscles and coordination all have the ability to change, so I want you to come away from this chapter with hope that you will once again be able to do the things you want to. Whether you're contending with tissue damage, nerve pain or a combination of both, as you move into Part 2, you'll come to see that there are lots of adaptations you can make to your daily life to strengthen and heal your back.

First, though, let's delve into the next chapter, which explores the different types of back pain.

CHAPTER 2

Types of Back Pain

NO MATTER HOW we feel about it, pain is a vital function that gives us a warning of potential or actual injury. As we'll explore, we experience pain physically, but we also experience it emotionally as it is affected by things such as fear, anxiety, past experiences of pain and even our beliefs around pain. Having a better understanding of this will help you to realise that, while pain can be complicated, we can take steps to change it.

In this chapter, we're going to explore the different types of pain so you can better understand what your amazing body is doing. My hope is that you'll then be armed with essential knowledge to enable you to understand your body's natural protection response, better describe your symptoms accurately when talking to your doctor and feel empowered to manage the specific kind of back pain you may be experiencing. Through the course of Part 2, you'll come to recognise that small adaptations to what you're doing daily will enable you to take control of your pain and therefore respond quicker to your body's natural healing response.

Let's start with the two main ways the body can interpret pain: nociceptive and neuropathic pain.

Nociceptive versus Neuropathic Pain

Nociceptive pain is caused by actual physical damage to the body, such as an injured bone or muscle, or injured skin from a cut or injection. The pain occurs when your nervous system reports this to your brain – it's the body's natural defence system against harmful actions.[1] This type of pain changes with movement or load – for example, a broken ankle will become more painful if you put weight on it.

Let's apply nociceptive pain down to a real-life situation. You have just woken up from a wonderful sleep and you get out of bed and sleepily walk to the bathroom, but accidentally step on a plug that was left on the floor when you were unpacking your work bag yesterday. (We have all been there, you are not alone.) When this happens, it usually goes something like this:

- You step on the plug.
- You quickly jump off the plug.
- You fall to the floor and use your hands to hold your foot (while screaming profanities).
- You then check your foot, looking for a gaping hole because that level of pain surely must have taken your entire foot off.
- The pain gradually calms down and you might be left with a bruise and soreness, but ultimately you get on with your day.

When you stand on the plug, the pain receptors (known as nociceptors) detect pain and the information is sent to the brain, where it is processed. Your brain then interprets it and decides whether or not to give you pain.

Nociceptive pain can also alert you to *potential* damage. For example, if you accidentally touch a hot surface, the immediate sharp pain serves as a warning to remove your hand swiftly, avoiding further injury.

Neuropathic pain, on the other hand, is the result of damage to the peripheral or central nervous system itself, and this can come from physical injury (such as nerve irritation), disease (such as multiple sclerosis) or following a stroke. It often feels like burning or shooting pain, but it can also be any type or quality of pain, and this type of pain most often leads to long-term pain as nervous system damage is more difficult to heal.[2] An example of neuropathic pain is the experience of someone recovering from a severe bout of shingles. This viral infection takes its toll on nerve cells, causing damage to the peripheral or central nervous system. This type of pain is remarkably diverse in its manifestations – it can feel like an intense burning or shooting sensation, akin to electric shocks, or extreme sensitivity to touch.

Alongside nociceptive and neuropathic pain, all of your past experiences and emotions are stored within your body, sort of like a vast library, and this emotional imprint can manifest in the form of pain, or influence the levels of pain in your body. If this sounds a bit woo-woo, I understand, but please stick with me.

How the brain can create pain

The brain can generate pain signals not only in response to tissue damage, but also in reaction to emotional and psychological symptoms. This intricate connection between the mind and pain is increased by conditions such as psychogenic pain. This is where emotional distress can manifest as physical discomfort as the anxiety that comes with being in pain only makes it worse.[3,4] For example, your brain might be conditioned to feel pain as soon as you sit at your desk, or when you are asked to do a particular movement in the gym, or every time you go and see a dentist. The brain goes into 'protection mode', and sometimes it can be a bit overprotective . . . Think of it like a super protective parent: it will give you pain when it doesn't need to, to stop you from doing something that it usually associates with feeling pain. The brain's interpretation of threat, stress or unresolved emotions can amplify pain experiences, creating a false reality that can be like tissue damage. It's so important to understand that pain isn't always a sign of structural harm, and all the steps in Part 2 will enable you to take back control and reduce your pain.

HOW YOUR ENVIRONMENT CAN IMPACT PAIN PERCEPTION

- Temperature: Cold temperatures may increase pain sensitivity, while warmth and heat may provide soothing pain relief.
- Noise levels: Loud or continuous noise can contribute to stress and increase pain sensitivity. White noise or calming music may promote relaxation.
- Surroundings and stress levels: High-stress environments can amplify pain severity, while supportive and stress-reducing environments can alleviate pain.

Remember, individual responses to these environmental factors may vary from person to person.

Acute Back Pain

This is the type of pain where you bend down to pick up a sock and you 'feel something go' (these are words I hear over and over again in clinic). This is usually followed by excruciating pain and the inability to move from that position or, in some cases, falling to the floor and being unable to move.

Often movement can cause a sharp, excruciating pain in every direction, and the pain may be specific to a particular location or it might travel to another location, for example, shooting pain down your leg or arm. This pain can be extremely scary and can be quite traumatic for people who have never experienced such intense pain before. It is easy to panic and start to believe that you might never be able to get up again! This is also known as pain catastrophising, which I will cover in Chapter 4.

Acute back pain is considered to be pain or discomfort that lasts fewer than six weeks, and it can be either nociceptive pain or pain created in the brain, as we explored above.

Naturally, the cause of acute back pain differs according to age. The older you are, the more likely it is the pain may be due to degenerative causes like osteoporosis, fractures, osteophytic growth (see osteophytes, page 17) or spinal stenosis (narrowing of the spinal canal). These changes that occur as you age are connected to your genetics. However, there are ways to prevent this from getting worse, such as weight-bearing exercises and resistance training, which we will cover in Chapter 3. Other common causes of acute pain that I see in my clinics range from sports injuries, sprains and dislocations to surgery and sleeping awkwardly.

Acute pain often serves as a warning sign and can be a signal to pause or modify our activities, so we can respond appropriately and potentially prevent more serious injuries or complications.

Acute back pain is scary but actually has promising improvement rates and usually gets better with non-invasive treatment. This is why the majority of times when someone experiences this kind of pain, it is unlikely that they will require an X-ray or an MRI.[5,6,7] There is also the risk that conducting an MRI may actually lead to finding a problem without there being any symptoms, which can have a detrimental impact on a person's perception of the strength of their back (see page 253 for more on this). As we saw in Chapter 1, imaging of the spine has a high chance of finding abnormalities in people with no symptoms (see page 20). Therefore it is advised that imaging only occurs in carefully selected people.[8]

'TECH NECK'

This is a term used to describe a type of neck pain that is caused by prolonged use of electronic devices such as smartphones, tablets and computers. The repeated use of these devices often leads to people craning their necks forwards and looking down for extended periods of time, which is thought to cause a sharp pain in the muscles or joints of the neck, and can often radiate to the back. Other common symptoms of tech neck include:

- Stiffness in the neck: This may make it difficult to turn your head or move your neck.
- Headaches: Particularly at the base of the skull.
- Shoulder pain: This may be aching or sharp and may be felt in the muscles or joints of the shoulders.
- Upper back pain: Particularly between the shoulder blades.
- Tingling or numbness: Prolonged pressure on the nerves in the neck can cause tingling or numbness in the arms, hands or fingers.

If these symptoms resonate with you, it's worth taking regular breaks from looking at your screen – maybe make a cup of tea or take a short walk if you have the ability to. Gentle movements like twisting in your chair and bending forwards and backwards can also improve the movement throughout your whole back, including your neck, and therefore relieve any aches or stiffness. The quick and easy desk mobility routine below is a great way to help with any pain as a result of tech neck.

Seated desk mobility routine

These three exercises are easy to do while sitting at your desk during the working day. It's great to do all of them, but if you feel one works better for you than another, feel free to pick and choose as you wish!

1. Neck and shoulder stretch:
   - Gently tilt your head to one side, bringing your ear towards your shoulder until you feel a stretch along the side of your neck.

- Hold the stretch for 10–15 seconds, breathing deeply.
- Repeat on the other side.
- Perform gentle neck circles by slowly and smoothly rotating your head clockwise for ten seconds and then counterclockwise for ten seconds.

2. Seated spinal twist:
   - Place your right hand on the outside of your left knee and your left hand on the back or arm of your chair.
   - Twist to the left, looking over your left shoulder.
   - Hold the twist for 10–15 seconds, feeling a gentle stretch through your spine.
   - Repeat on the other side.

3. Seated leg extensions with ankle circles:
   - Extend one leg straight out in front of you, flexing your foot.
   - Hold the extended position for 5–10 seconds, feeling a stretch in your hamstring.
   - Rotate your ankle clockwise for five seconds and then counterclockwise for five seconds.
   - Perform this sequence 2–3 times for each leg.

COCCYX PAIN

Also known as pain in your butt, coccyx pain is really common. So many people experience discomfort there, but they're often embarrassed or worried to tell anyone or seek advice or treatment. Some common symptoms include:

- Pain at the base of your spine when sitting down.
- Pain at the base of your spine when getting up from sitting.
- Pain or an ache at the base of your spine that comes and goes or stays there constantly.

The good news is that 90 per cent of coccyx pain is reduced by methods that aren't invasive.[9] The following aids may help:

- A coccyx cushion to soften the surface you are sitting on and help the coccyx heal itself. This can be particularly helpful for those who have seated jobs.
- Anti-inflammatories to reduce inflammation.
- Exercises and mobility drills to strengthen around the coccyx.

Chronic Back Pain

This is the kind of pain that you've had for a longer period of time, usually 12 weeks or more. It can involve changes in the nervous system, which can contribute to ongoing pain even after the initial injury or condition has healed. Chronic pain is continuous and people often worry that it's never going to end. It can range from things like sciatica to a dull ache in your lower back or an ongoing pain in the mid-back. My clients often end up describing it as pain that they have 'just got used to' – like something they have in the background as a dull nagging ache that occasionally becomes more obvious, and it fluctuates on a day-to-day basis. Chronic pain can be either nociceptive or neuropathic pain.

The all-encompassing nature of chronic pain can be attributed to its effects on various aspects of a person's life. Pain signals can disrupt normal sensory processing, making it difficult to concentrate on everyday tasks and interfering with cognitive functioning. The constant presence of pain can also lead to sleep disturbances, fatigue and emotional distress, further exacerbating the impact on daily activities and overall quality of life.

Chronic back pain can also be worrying and can often lead to the unhealthy spiral of a negative mindset and fear-based life restrictions. This is essentially when you are too scared to partake in activities you enjoy as you are worried they may cause your pain to flare up or get worse. This can also then result in more negative thinking and lead to poor mental health by keeping yourself from activities you might enjoy. We'll explore this more fully in Chapter 4.

All the steps in Part 2 will show you how small adaptations can have a big impact on your chronic pain.

EASY WAYS TO MANAGE CHRONIC PAIN

Each individual is different. However, some ways in which you can take steps to manage chronic pain are:

- Try to get around 7–8 hours' sleep a night.
- Drink more water.
- Practise mindfulness for just ten minutes a day.
- Keep moving, even if it's just a gentle walk or vacuuming the house.

We'll cover all of the above in more detail in Part 2.

Non-specific Back Pain

I know this is a bit annoying – it sounds wishy-washy, right? Essentially, non-specific back pain means that you are experiencing pain that has no specific cause, such as tissue damage or an underlying disease. Most back pain is non-specific back pain.

Non-specific back pain can sometimes be referred to as 'simple back pain', which I'm not a fan of as it can sound quite patronising and actually there is nothing 'simple' about pain.

Non-specific back pain is essentially neuropathic pain – and it is complicated. According to the World Health Organization (WHO), risk factors include low physical activity levels, smoking, obesity and high physical stress at work.[10]

If you are not sure what is causing your back pain and think it may be non-specific, I want to reassure you that the steps in Part 2 will still give you the tools to quickly be able to help yourself and reduce your pain.

Nerve Root Pain

Nerve pain often manifests as unusual sensations, such as burning, tingling, stabbing or electric shock-like sensations. These occur because the damaged nerves are sending unusual signals to the brain. If you have pain that seems to travel or that you feel in more than one place, it may indeed be nerve root pain – but it may also not be this at all. Nerve root pain is also described as 'radiculopathy', which is when you have pain in multiple areas. Pain can radiate to other areas of the back – for example, people will experience lower back pain and then also feel pain or pins and needles down the leg. This is often referred to as sciatica (see below).[11]

WHAT IS SCIATICA?

Sciatica is an inflammation of the sciatic nerve and symptoms include:

- weakness in the leg or foot
- numbness or pins and needles in the foot
- pain down the leg, as a dull ache or a sharp, shooting pain

Sciatica varies from mild discomfort to constant agony. There are many causes of sciatica and it's important that these are diagnosed by a musculoskeletal expert. Sciatica can be aided when the correct diagnosis is given, and with the correct treatment and rehabilitation.

If you're really struggling right now with sciatica, know that you are not alone and that your body is really strong . . . you just need a little guidance.

Symptoms are often felt in a number of ways, and this can also be down to how the individual describes their pain. I might describe it as shooting pain, while someone else would say it is sharp pain, but it essentially means the same thing. The most common descriptive words I hear in clinic are 'tingling', 'pins and needles', 'ants crawling on my skin', 'shooting pain', 'weakness' or simply 'pain'.

Nerve pain is normally due to compression of the nerve where it comes out of the spine. It usually occurs as a second symptom to a primary cause such as:

- disc degenerative disease
- facet joint degeneration
- spondylolisthesis
- ligament hypertrophy
- osteoarthritis

The most common areas in which people experience nerve root pain are the neck (cervical) area or the lower back (lumbar) region. It isn't so common in the middle of your back (thoracic).[12] Excessive movement might increase the risk of nerve compression or irritation. Since the thoracic spine has less mobility, there may be a lower likelihood of nerve-related problems due to movement-related issues.

You can also get this nerve pain from a trauma like lifting something heavy without properly bracing your body for it and adopting the correct form (we've all been there – see page 53 for guidance on a proper lifting technique) or being in a car accident – if it's a minor bump, this can give you whiplash and lead to nerve-related pain. It is uncommon, but there are also conditions like diabetes that can cause a lack of blood flow and consequently cause nerve root pain.

WHERE DOES NERVE ROOT PAIN GO?

The symptoms and where you might experience nerve pain depend on which of the nerves are affected. It's a bit like your spine is the main circuit board for all the houses on the street and then it splits to power each individual house:

- The neck: This area provides power and feeling to your upper body and down your arms.
- The mid-back: This area provides movement, feeling and power to your torso, abdomen and the muscles of the chest like your pecs.
- The lower back: This area provides movement, power and feeling to the lower back, glutes, legs and feet.

When you see a musculoskeletal expert like an osteopath, they have the knowledge to understand from your symptoms where your pain is coming from and even what exact nerve or vertebra that pain is coming from according to where you feel the pain.

There are tests that can be done to find out if there is an impingement or compression of the nerve at the spine. Two common tests I do in clinic that you may be able to do at home are:

1. Straight leg raise (SLR) test
   - Purpose: The SLR test can help assess whether there is compression or irritation of the sciatic nerve (which runs down the back of each leg), which can sometimes be caused by lower back nerve irritation.
   - Procedure:
     1. Lie on your back with your legs straight.
     2. Slowly lift one leg off the ground while keeping it straight. Try to raise it as high as you can.
     3. Note any pain, tingling or numbness you feel, especially in the lower back, buttocks or down the leg.

- Interpretation: If you experience radiating pain, tingling or numbness that follows a specific nerve pathway during this test, it may indicate sciatic nerve compression or irritation. However, this test alone cannot determine the exact cause or location of the impingement.

2. Resisted hip flexion
    - Purpose: Resisted hip flexion is used to assess potential issues with the femoral nerve, helping to identify discomfort or weakness in the front of the thigh. Lower back pain with femoral neuritis (nerve inflammation) is quite common.[13]
    - Procedure:
        1. While seated or lying down, attempt to lift one leg straight up off the ground.
        2. Apply gentle resistance with your hands, pushing your thigh downwards.
        3. Pay attention to any pain, discomfort or weakness in the front of the thigh during the movement.
    - Interpretation: If you experience pain or weakness in the front of the thigh during resisted hip flexion, it could indicate problems with the femoral nerve. However, this self-assessment is not a definitive diagnosis, and any concerning symptoms should be discussed with a healthcare professional for a more thorough evaluation.

Although nerve pain can be extremely worrying, it's highly likely that you don't need to be concerned. Nerve root pain is rarely caused by anything serious and studies have shown that the steps in Part 2 can contribute to positive outcomes with this type of pain.[14] By adopting this multidirectional plan, the majority of patients I see in clinic improve significantly.

PROPER LIFTING TECHNIQUE

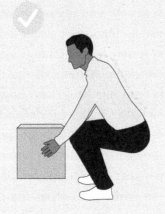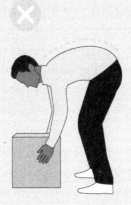

- Think about the amount of load to be lifted. If the weight is too heavy for one person, wait until someone can help you.
- Bend your knees to lower the body to the level of the item being lifted.
- Keep your feet shoulder width apart to ensure a stable base.
- Keep your back straight.
- Use a firm grip.
- Keep the weight close to your body.
- Point your feet in the direction of movement. Never rotate your back while lifting at the same time.
- Lift using your legs, rather than the muscles in your back.

Referred Pain

This is when you experience pain in an area of your body that is not the cause of it. This could be sciatic pain, when you may have a pinched nerve at the spinal level but feel the pain down the sciatic nerve in the leg, or referred pain from organs.

Now, I know this sounds scary. When anyone mentions the fact that an organ can cause us physical pain, it can be worrying and we often fear that it may be something sinister. However, I'm going to take you through some of the most common organs that refer pain into our backs and how it's actually the same as the warning light on your car dashboard. If we stop and think about it for a minute, it's actually pretty clever that our body is telling us that something is wrong or needs attention, regardless of whether it is serious or not.

Visceral pain (organ pain) is when pain from the deep organs is felt in the surrounding joints or muscles. There are a few different theories on which organs refer to which location, but they tend to be very close to the vicinity in which the pain is felt.[15]

One example of how our organs can warn us if there is an issue is if we are constipated. This is not healthy for our digestive system, so our intestine sends pain to our lower back and stomach. Another example is when we have pain in the lower stomach due to a bladder infection. Of course, there are also the more well-known conditions of kidney stones or infection causing pain in the lower back (along with other symptoms that may include a fever or burning sensation during urination). There is also the sharp pain you feel on the lower right side of your abdomen if you have appendicitis and,

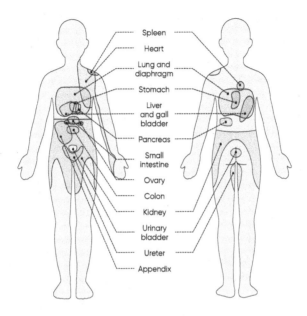

Spleen

Heart

Lung and diaphragm

Stomach

Liver and gall bladder

Pancreas

Small intestine

Ovary

Colon

Kidney

Urinary bladder

Ureter

Appendix

again, this is our body's way of telling us we need to get it sorted urgently to avoid a more serious emergency. We can also often get back pain or joint pain when there are medical emergencies like a heart condition or heart attack. This can present as pain in the centre of your chest and down your arm.

IRENE

Irene came to see me with pain in her lower back that she had had for three to four weeks. She explained that she works as a teacher and is on her feet and active from around 7.30am until 6pm most days. She explained that the pain in her back was like a dull ache and it had gradually become more and more intense recently. She wanted to seek out an osteopath as, in her words, 'lower back pain runs in my family'.

On examination, there were no real structural worries and I asked her how much water she drank every day. Irene said she drank three glasses a day, which was better than some but not great. I then asked her how many times she was able to visit the toilet at work. She said that most of the time she just holds it in till she gets home, by which point she is desperate and has to run to the loo.

I decided to examine Irene for a kidney infection (there is a technique osteopaths can do to see if it causes pain). This test came back positive and so I explained that I didn't think it was her back and that actually she needed to see her GP to have a urine sample taken as she might have a urine or kidney infection.

After a few weeks, Irene called to say she was feeling much better. She did have blood in her urine when the GP tested it and she was given antibiotics for her infection. Her back pain had disappeared!

This is a good example of how back pain can be caused by visceral organs and be telling us that something needs to be sorted out.

Another great example of referred pain is, of course, menstrual pain in women. When a woman is experiencing their period each month they often complain of lower abdominal pain, lower back pain and can experience headaches and achy legs. All of this is as a result of hormones that can impact our sleep, stress levels and the way in which our brain thinks about pain. Also, because a woman's uterus is physically shedding its lining and, in order to do this, it needs to contract, this might cause pain in the stomach and lower back.

PERIOD BACK PAIN EXERCISES

Many women experience lower back pain when they have their period. Quite often it's tempting to lie in bed with a hot water bottle and not move during this time. However, research has shown that engaging in movement may reduce your pain symptoms.[16] This movement does not need to be strenuous; as you'll come to see in Chapter 3, movement can also be slow and controlled.

The exercises below have helped to relieve my symptoms and have also helped many of my patients in clinic.

- Child's pose: Kneel on the floor, then sit back on your heels and lower your upper body forwards, extending your arms in front of you. Hold for 30 seconds while focusing on deep breathing.
- Knee tuck and rock: Lie on your back and bend both your knees. Bring your knees to your chest and interlace your fingers behind your thighs. Gently rock from side to side with your knees tucked in.
- Cobra stretch: Lie on your front, place your hands out in front of you and extend your back backwards like a cobra.
- Seated twist: Sit cross-legged on the floor or on a chair with your right leg over your left. Bring your left hand to your right knee, sit up tall and twist round to your right and stretch. Repeat on the other side.

All of these stretches should be held for 20–30 seconds. Repeat as you feel necessary. I also recommend going for a walk to help ease symptoms of pain in your lower back.

If you're concerned that your back pain may be referred pain from elsewhere in the body, please see a medical professional for a proper diagnosis. The steps in Part 2, especially keep moving and sleep better, may also help to alleviate your pain.

Risk Factors for Back Pain

Identifying the characteristics that predict who is at risk of developing back pain is beneficial for the prevention and treatment of it. Risk factors for general back pain include:

- Lack of exercise.
- Age: Back pain most commonly occurs for the first time in people between the ages of 30 and 50.[17]
- Obesity: Excess weight can lead to an increased chance of having back pain.
- Smoking: There is some research to show that smokers are more likely to have back pain.[18]
- Stress and anxiety: We will discuss this in detail in Chapter 4.

One of the most common types of back pain that I see in my clinics is lower back pain, and this is mirrored across the world. In 2020, global instances of lower back pain impacted 619 million people, and projections suggest a rise to 843 million cases by 2050. This surge is primarily attributed to population growth and an ageing demographic.[19]

Lower back pain stands as the primary cause of disability worldwide and it is a condition that can manifest at any point in a person's lifespan; nearly everyone encounters lower back pain at least once. According to the WHO, the frequency of lower back pain occurrence escalates with advancing age, peaking at around 80 years, with the highest density of cases arising within the 50–55-year age bracket.[20] The most prevalent form of lower back pain is categorised as non-specific back pain, making up around 90 per cent of all cases.

One of the risk factors for chronic lower back pain that has been consistently replicated in multiple studies is increasing age. Additionally, previous back pain, job dissatisfaction and pain below the knee have also been identified as predictors of chronic lower back pain.[21,22,23] Depression has been noted to be associated with various chronic pain syndromes, and its relationship with chronic back pain in particular has been consistently reported in multiple studies.[24]

Women are more commonly affected by lower back pain than men, and some studies suggest that they are also more likely to develop chronic lower back pain. Other factors that have been linked to the development of chronic lower back pain include high levels of psychological stress, low levels of physical activity, obesity and lack of good-quality sleep.[25]

Whether you have one, two or more of the risk factors mentioned above, it's important to remember that pain is not straightforward and is often a complex and multidimensional experience. Below are a few reasons why pain can be challenging to understand and manage:

1. Subjectivity: Pain is a subjective experience, meaning it is influenced by an individual's unique perception, emotions, beliefs and past experiences. What may be painful for one person might not be as painful for another.
2. Multifactorial nature: Pain can be influenced by various factors, including physical, psychological, social and environmental. These factors can interact and amplify

or diminish the pain experience, making it difficult to pinpoint a single cause or solution.

3. Sensitisation: In some cases, the nervous system can become sensitised, leading to heightened pain sensitivity or the perception of pain, even in the absence of an obvious injury or pathology (see page 120).

4. Individual variability: Each person's pain experience is unique, and what works for one individual may not work for another. The effectiveness of pain management strategies can vary from person to person, highlighting the need for personalised approaches.

Back Exercises

Back pain is not just one type of pain, but rather a complex experience that people feel in different ways. Often with back pain, it's also not uncommon for things to get a bit tangled. Sometimes, you might find yourself dealing with both nociceptive and neuropathic pain – tissue damage *and* nerve pain – simultaneously. Alternatively, it might be that your brain is perceiving pain based on a previous traumatic experience. Pain is a complex phenomenon influenced by various factors, and its management often requires a multipronged approach, which the four steps in Part 2 aim to provide.

Before we move on to getting a diagnosis for your pain, I'd like you to ask yourself the following questions:

1. What type of pain described above most resonates with you?

2. Can you identify a specific cause for your pain or is it non-specific?

Your answers should empower you to feel more confident when speaking to health professionals about your pain and may also give you the ability to get an accurate diagnosis.

We'll cover the benefits of exercise for back pain thoroughly in Chapter 3, but for now, here are some exercises for specific areas of the back to help you get started on easing your pain. If you're experiencing any niggles or twinges in your back, you should try to do these exercises three times a day. Being slow and controlled is key here.

Mid-back pain exercises

Try these two simple exercises if you experience pain in the middle of your back:

1. Dumbbell hold: Hold two light weights out in front of you with your arms straight for as long as you can. Check for any tension in your neck, and make sure your shoulders are soft and not reaching up to your ears.
2. Extension: Lie on your front and come up onto your elbows. Pause and repeat.

Lower back pain exercises

Below are some great exercises for lower back pain:

- Alternate leg and arm raises: On all fours, lift up your left arm and right leg and then right arm and left leg. Repeat this 20 times, or within your limits.
- Back extensions: Lie down on your front. Using your arms and keeping your hips on the floor, gently push up into a lower-level extension of your lower back. If you

can, try to go into a full arm extension, keeping your hips on the floor. Hold for 20 seconds and repeat three times.

- Glute bridges: My favourite. Lie on your back with your knees bent. Slowly lift up your pelvis and squeeze your bottom at the top. Hold for 30 seconds and repeat three times.

One-sided lower back pain exercises

Have you ever felt like one side of your lower back was quite sore? One exercise that works well with my patients is clam shells:

- With a band or scarf tied tightly around your thighs, lie on your side and prop yourself up with your elbow. Then gently bring your knees apart, keeping your feet pressed together. Avoid rolling your hips back, and keep your pelvis upright. The band or scarf around your thighs will act as resistance.
- If you want to try to push this further, you can also go into a side plank and add clam shells.

Take this one step at a time and always start with the standard clam shells first.

Pain when you bend forwards exercises

- cobra stretch (see page 57)
- glute bridges (see above)
- seated cat-camel (see page 104)

For all these exercises, your rep range is dependent on when you feel that muscle contract and burn slightly. For some that might be five reps and for others it might be 20. Note: These exercises aren't always beneficial for everyone. If any of these make you feel sore or worse, please stop and seek advice from your osteopath or GP.

WHEN TO CONSULT A HEALTHCARE PROVIDER FOR BACK PAIN

- Duration: If your back pain persists for more than a few weeks despite home treatment and self-care.
- Intensity: When the pain is agony and does not improve with rest or adapting your activities.
- Radiation: If the pain spreads down a leg or both legs, especially if it goes below the knee.
- Neurological symptoms: If the pain is accompanied by muscle weakness, numbness or tingling in one or both legs, which impacts your ability to walk.
- Concerning signs: If back pain is also accompanied by unexplained weight loss.

WHEN TO SEEK URGENT MEDICAL ATTENTION FOR BACK PAIN

- Bowel or bladder control: If you lose control of your bladder or bowel completely.
- Fever: If back pain is accompanied by a high fever.
- Trauma: Following a big fall, blow to the back or accident, emergency medical attention is crucial.

Getting a Diagnosis

Experiencing pain without a clear diagnosis or apparent cause can be frustrating and challenging. Hopefully, you'll also have recognised that some or all of your symptoms are extremely common, and so please know that you are not alone. I'm hoping this chapter has offered you some reassurance on how complex pain is and how everything you are experiencing is completely valid.

I've included some tips below on how to get a diagnosis and what to do if you're not satisfied with your initial evaluation:

1. Seek medical attention: Schedule an appointment with a healthcare professional, such as your primary care physician or a specialist, to discuss your symptoms and concerns. Osteopaths, physiotherapists and other healthcare professionals undergo extensive training to be able to conduct thorough examinations when it comes to pain and recognising the cause of this pain.

2. Describe the pain you're experiencing in detail: I've included some tips below on communicating your pain. Try to mention any accompanying symptoms or patterns you've noticed.

3. Keep a pain diary: Document your pain episodes, including the intensity, duration and any triggers or patterns you observe. Note any activities or factors that may aggravate or alleviate the pain. This information can be helpful for your healthcare provider in identifying potential causes or patterns over time.

4. Advocate for yourself: If you're not satisfied with the initial evaluation or the provided explanations, don't hesitate to seek a second opinion. It's important to find a healthcare provider who listens to your concerns and takes them seriously.

5. Explore alternative therapies: In addition to conventional medical treatments, you might consider complementary or alternative therapies, such as acupuncture or mindfulness practices. These approaches can sometimes provide relief or help manage pain. We'll explore treatment options in Chapter 7 so you can decide what might be right for you.

6. Practise self-care: While searching for answers, it's crucial to take care of your overall well-being using the four steps outlined in Part 2. Engage in stress-reducing activities like meditation, deep breathing exercises or gentle physical activities, as stress can sometimes exacerbate pain symptoms. Adequate sleep, a balanced diet and regular exercise can also contribute to your overall health and potentially improve pain management.

7. Seek support: Dealing with unexplained pain can be emotionally and mentally challenging. Consider reaching out to a support group or therapist who specialises in chronic pain or pain management. They can offer guidance, coping strategies and emotional support during your journey. (See also the Useful Resources on page 275.)

Remember, these suggestions are not a substitute for professional medical advice.

How to communicate about your pain

When you go to a healthcare professional – whether that is your local doctor, a physiotherapist, osteopath or reiki healer – it can be tough to verbalise what is going on with your pain. Often, they ask you questions that you've never even thought about and it can be difficult to describe your pain. Sometimes this can confuse you and almost make you feel a bit silly: 'How can I not describe my pain when it is my body? This is so embarrassing.'

Firstly, it is not embarrassing! Healthcare professionals are used to helping their patients communicate and it's totally normal not to know how to describe your pain. If a healthcare professional ever makes you feel inadequate for not knowing how to communicate your pain, or any health concern for that matter, it might be worth seeking a second opinion or requesting an alternative practitioner, if possible.

Understanding how to communicate your pain is worth it for several reasons:

1. Accurate diagnosis: When you can communicate your pain effectively, doctors and other healthcare professionals can better understand the nature and severity of your symptoms. This can help them make a more accurate diagnosis.

2. Proper treatment: Being able to communicate your pain can also help ensure that you receive appropriate treatment. This can include pain management strategies, medication, physical therapy or other interventions that can help alleviate your symptoms and improve your quality of life.

3. Empowerment: Communicating your pain can help you feel more empowered and in control of your healthcare. When you can express your concerns and needs clearly, you can collaborate with your healthcare team to develop a treatment plan that works for you.

4. Emotional well-being: Pain can have a significant impact on emotional well-being. When you are able to express your pain and be heard, it can help reduce feelings of isolation and increase feelings of support and validation.

Below are some examples of how you might describe your pain and the information that we, as professionals, want to know to get to the cause of what is going on. Some questions they may ask you and some example answers include:

- What is the location of your pain?

Example answer: 'I have a sharp pain in my lower back that radiates down my right leg.'

- How would you describe the quality of your pain?

Example answer: 'It feels like a burning sensation that is constant and intensifies when I sit for long periods of time.'

- How severe is your pain?

Example answer: 'On a scale of 1–10, it's about an 8, and it's been consistently at this level for the past few days.'

- What triggers your pain or makes it worse?

Example answer: 'Sitting or standing for long periods of time, bending over or lifting heavy objects seem to make my pain worse.'

- How does the pain affect your daily life?

Example answer: 'I have trouble sleeping at night, I can't sit or stand for long periods of time and I've had to take time off work because of the pain.'

- Have you tried any pain relief methods and, if so, how effective were they?

Example answer: 'I've tried taking over-the-counter pain medication and using heat and ice, but they haven't provided much relief.'

- How would you describe your emotional response to the pain?

Example answer: 'I feel frustrated and worried that the pain will never go away, and it's impacting my ability to enjoy life.'

I've listed below some common words that you might find useful when thinking about how your pain actually feels. Circle the ones that are most relevant to you:

- dull ache
- sharp pain
- constant
- it comes and goes
- electric
- it moves around
- worse in the morning
- worse at night
- no pattern at all
- itchy feeling
- numb
- heavy
- compressed
- pain that travels around the body

Using some of these words is a great way to initiate a conversation with your doctor or osteopath about how you're feeling.

PAIN IN THE WORKPLACE

Most of us spend the majority of our time at work, so, as well as speaking to a health professional about your back pain, having open communication with your manager and other stakeholders can help your stress levels and, believe it or not, also help pain in the workplace. This can include having regular meetings, feedback sessions and open-door policies.

In fact, workplace culture as a whole is growing in importance. Creating a positive work environment by promoting work–life balance, providing a comfortable and safe workplace and promoting wellness initiatives can all help employees feel supported and less stressed, which has a positive impact on pain.

While medical findings and diagnoses are undeniably crucial, they represent just one facet of the complex landscape of health and back pain. It's equally vital to consider the multitude of other factors that can influence back pain, such as lifestyle, stress and mental health. The steps that follow are full of practical tips, strategies and tricks that have proven to be effective with my clients in multiple situations. Whether you're dealing with acute pain, seeking long-term solutions to secure your back for the future or are currently waiting for back surgery, these insights will be your trusted companions on your healing journey. By adopting the tools and strategies outlined in the four steps, you can take a more well-rounded approach to managing and alleviating your back pain. Following these steps will also aid in a smoother recovery journey after surgery. It's worth exploring these insights, as they may introduce new advice and practices that you may not have considered before, and also encourage a deeper understanding of the intricate relationship between physical and emotional well-being.

PART 2

Let the Healing Begin

Welcome to the second part of your journey towards a healthier, stronger back. In this section, we'll dive deep into the tools and techniques that will empower you with the knowledge and skills necessary to take control of and heal your back – for life.

Remember, there is no quick fix for back pain. Instead, these steps are about making manageable, gradual changes that, in time, will create long-lasting habits and the beginning of a new relationship with your pain. You might notice a difference after just a couple of weeks, or it might take a few months; our bodies all respond differently and that's OK. The most important thing is that you take things at your own pace.

However, as I mentioned in the Introduction, if you can try to embed at least one new tool a week from each step, and make a commitment to adopt these strategies in the long term, it will really make a difference to your pain. Though I understand that healing your back is not a one-size-fits-all endeavour, for those of you who prefer more structured guidance, there are some weekly plans at the end of each step (see pages 112, 146, 184 and 220).

Ultimately, my mission is to instil in you a renewed sense of confidence, not just in your back's immediate well-being, but in its long-term strength and resilience. The client stories shared in this section are a testament to the transformative power of perseverance, making informed choices and a deep commitment to personal well-being. I hope you will feel inspired by them and make a similar pledge to take small steps to heal your back.

It's time to turn the page on your back pain.

CHAPTER 3

Step 1: Keep Moving

WELCOME TO THE first step in your journey to healing your back. In this chapter, I will be covering not only the importance of movement when it comes to back pain, but also some reasons that may resonate with you about why you feel limited, and why it may not be as simple as 'moving more'. I will then explore the benefits of various exercises, such as swimming, running, strength training and stretching, so you can see what feels right for you.

We all know that our body takes time to adapt and the best way to introduce exercise into your day is slowly and consistently; I think it's fair to say that we don't expect to go to the gym once and lose 5kg. Therefore, once you've read through the different options and identified which exercise(s) you'd like to try, start by incorporating at least ten minutes three times a week, before gradually building up to 30 minutes of moderate-intensity exercise four or five times a week, though always working within your own limits. There is also a weekly plan on page 112 to help guide you through incorporating movement into your daily life gradually.

Most of the suggestions in this step are doable at home without the need for any special equipment or a gym membership, but if you want to engage in the mobility or strength exercises, you might find it more comfortable to do so on an exercise mat. As you build up your strength, you may also want to invest in some weights or a kettlebell, but this is not essential as your body weight is often enough to build up muscle mass and strength.

Once you've read about all the benefits of exercise and are ready to get started with incorporating some small changes into your daily life, make sure you complete the goal-setting exercise on page 106, taking the time to define your goals and establish what you really want to get out of this step. Don't forget to also fill in the progress tracker on page 113 every week, so you can gauge your progress with this step and see how far you have come.

(As always, consult with a healthcare professional before starting any exercise programme, especially if you have an existing back condition. They can provide guidance and ensure you choose exercises that are safe and suitable for your specific needs.)

Movement Is Medicine

Most of us know that exercise is good for us. We've been told for years that it can help to reduce the risk of illnesses such as cardiovascular disease, stroke, type 2 diabetes and some cancers, and being physically active can also help to boost your mood, self-esteem and sleep quality, as well as reduce your risk of stress and clinical depression.[1]

The number of studies conducted on the long-term health benefits of physical activity is vast. One study that looked at more than 250,000 participants showed that there are clear, positive, long-term benefits from regular physical activity for conditions such as obesity, coronary heart disease, type 2 diabetes, Alzheimer's and dementia.[2]

Moreover, when it comes specifically to the impact of movement and pain levels, physical movement, in whatever shape or form that may be, has been proven to reduce pain, whatever your age. Physical activity and exercise is guaranteed to reduce the severity of pain and the ability to physically move, and consequently improve your quality of life. Research shows that most levels of activity and exercise can be beneficial in reducing pain and increasing the range of motion and functionality for people with muscular pain.[3] Those who have had major surgery for back pain or who suffer from medical conditions like osteoporosis have also shown big improvements in their pain levels due to movement.

In my clinics, I see people who have tried all sorts of things to help their level of pain. These range from invasive treatments, such as injections or surgery, to more holistic therapies, such as reiki or reflexology. Though in my opinion there is nothing wrong with any of these approaches and I respect all of them in their own right, the one consistent piece of advice that rings true is: physical movement is repeatedly proven to help reduce pain levels. In fact, a whopping 52.5 per cent of people experience relief from back pain through exercise.[4] So, it's time to bid farewell to those nagging aches and discover the transformative power of movement. You should begin your journey into exercise because it:

1. Strengthens your spine: Engaging in regular exercise, especially activities that target your core muscles, helps to build a strong foundation for your spine.
2. Increases flexibility and mobility: Incorporating stretching and flexibility exercises into your routine may help with

tight muscles, improve joint mobility and reduce pressure on your back.

3. Releases those feel-good endorphins: Movement is a natural painkiller. Physical activity triggers the release of endorphins, your body's feel-good chemicals, which can help reduce pain perception and elevate your mood.

Barriers to Exercise

From generation to generation, exercise has become trendier and better researched. And yet so many of us are still resistant to physical movement. The fear of pain or injury may in itself be a blockage to starting your movement journey, but I'm hoping this chapter will enable you to feel more confident.

There are many other barriers to exercise, which we'll explore below. You might find that some of these resonate with you.

Previous psychological trauma

It's sometimes hard to remember, but being picked 'last' for netball or football, or being considered 'bad' at sport and therefore being unpopular or picked on at school, can lead to long-term psychological trauma around exercise. This can create fear and a lack of motivation to get involved in any form of exercise.

This isn't limited to school sports; it can also be down to other childhood traumas (such as being shouted at by your parents), panic attacks or anxiety, which typically involve an increase in heart rate ('tachycardia' in medical lingo). There have been some instances where my patients have realised that their fear of exercise that involves cardio or an increased heart rate is down to associations with childhood memories of when they may have felt vulnerable or at risk. This usually relates to a childhood that may have contained major accidents, abuse in their home or bullying at school.

The fix: Recognise these connections and maybe seek professional help via the NHS or with a therapist to work through these past experiences. (See Useful Resources, page 275, for some organisations you could reach out to.)

Lack of time

Kids, work, social commitments, family events . . . these can all be extremely time-consuming. It can sometimes feel impossible even to think about how a workout could be fitted into your day – especially when you have young children and they are so dependent on you.

The fix: Try to incorporate movement into your daily life. This might be parking your car further away from the train station, getting off the bus one stop early, walking to the supermarket or taking the stairs instead of the lift. It can even look like some simple squats while waiting for the kettle to boil, or balancing/hopping on alternate legs while brushing your teeth. Even getting involved with your kids and playing with them is a great means of moving your body in ways you didn't think were still possible.

Lack of support

Another common barrier might be the people closest to you. This is often hard to admit as they are also the people you love and care for the most. But they may have their own opinions on movement or exercise and consequently feel quite opinionated about your choices.

The fix: Try to join a group exercise session or surround yourself with like-minded people. You may find that you have someone you work with or a neighbour who is often out running or goes to a Pilates class each week. Maybe you could ask to join them to see if it's something that you also enjoy. Try to ignore the naysayers and surround yourself with your biggest champions. If the naysayers are those who are close to you, they will understand that you want to change your life for the better.

Motivation and tiredness

We all feel this at different times in our lives. Sometimes it can be super hard to find the motivation to get up in the morning and do some exercise. In fact, it might be super hard just to get up, full stop.

The fix: Have an earlier night and get your exercise clothes (or your gym bag) ready for the next morning. You can also tell other people that you are going to do some exercise tomorrow, whether that is going for a walk, to a Pilates class or even arranging to meet one of your friends at the gym so that you have accountability. I personally like to exercise first thing in the morning – this means that it's done and dusted, and how the rest of my day pans out won't impact my workout.

TIPS FOR A WORKOUT MINDSET

Do you struggle to get into a workout mindset? Here are some ways that help me:

- Go with a friend: Accountability is the best.
- Create an epic playlist: Find your most inspiring tunes.
- Try a repetitive mantra: Count down from ten and then back up again while doing cardio, instead of focusing on how long is left.
- Think of someone you admire: What would they do? Would they get up and go to the gym?

Fear of injury

This is obviously what I see the most in clinic. It is one of the most common reasons by far that people don't want to implement movement or exercise into their life. This can often be due to a person injuring their back when doing a particular sport or exercise – for example, 'I was deadlifting in the gym and my back went into spasm' or 'I went to a yoga class and I turned awkwardly and was in agony for a week.' Often these narratives blame the exercise that was being engaged in at the time and consequently this creates fear around doing that particular activity or other similar activities again.

Remember, you injured your back in the gym; the gym didn't injure your back.

The fix: If you can, try to change your narrative by journalling each evening before bed. Writing down 'my body is strong' repeatedly and maybe saying it out loud can help to change your mindset around your fear. If this doesn't resonate with you, it may be worth seeking advice from your GP or health professional – they have the knowledge to be able to reassure you on what you should be trying to do when it comes to implementing movement in your daily life. This reassurance may help the fear that is associated with movement after having a traumatic injury or painful event. Taking small steps back into exercise can also reassure you that the pain won't be triggered again. For example, if you're used to lifting 50kg, start with 10kg and gradually build yourself back up. The tips and strategies in Step 2 (page 115) may also help you to change your mindset around pain.

OSTEO TOP TIP

We live in a world where we are expected to always move forwards and progress upwards. The truth is that there's nothing wrong with having to go back to basics and relearn something. When it comes to exercise, for example, it's OK to go back to the gym and start lifting weights that are lighter than you're used to lifting – it's definitely not a step backwards.

HANNAH

Hannah came into the clinic feeling very anxious about her lower back pain. She wasn't in pain when she came in,

---

but had experienced two extreme episodes of lower back pain, one of which involved her having to be taken into A&E and given strong painkillers. Naturally, these events were extremely traumatic for her and consequently she was fearful of treatment, exercise or anything new.

On examination, I noticed that when I asked Hannah to perform movements with her body, like bending forwards or backwards, or rotating, she did them very tentatively and moved a bit like she was a robot. However, when I put my hands on her back and asked her to do the same movements, she was able to exhibit more than double the range of movement, *without* pain. I didn't mention this to Hannah at first, and instead just said how great her movement felt. At the end of the session I noticed she had more confidence in her back and she was able to turn slightly further on her own, but not much.

I gave Hannah a simple rotation exercise to do every day at her desk and at home to encourage movement. By doing this each day, she was able to track her movement improving and also focus on how far she could see objects behind her. Even though this seems simple, when you fear movement, even just rotating further each day can be all it takes to give yourself some confidence.

Hannah is a classic example of how fear of injury can mean that your brain limits your movement. Her body was too scared to move on its own, but she felt reassured when I was moving her back for her. It was about retraining the brain.

Hannah would subsequently come into clinic and say things like, 'Goodness, I managed to lift the sofa with my husband and hoover and I didn't even think about my back pain.' This is how a change in the narrative can happen without you even realising.

If any of these barriers resonate with you, please know that you're not alone. There are many reasons why people are averse to physical movement, but, hopefully, by the end of this chapter you'll be inspired to incorporate it into your life once you understand the benefits it can bring to your overall health and, most importantly, your pain.

MYTH-BUSTER: REST ISN'T REHAB

This is an old one, but I still have clients who come in and say that if something hurts, they should stop completely. Bed rest is very much a thing of the past. If you injured yourself, it was once commonly thought that you needed to immobilise the joint or bone. However, surgeons now won't put a cast on a broken bone if they don't have to. In fact, they've found that you may heal faster if you aren't immobilised.[5] Those who have been in a car accident and have whiplash are no longer given a collar to wear and are encouraged to move their neck as much as possible to help them heal more quickly.[6] In addition, acute, sharp lower back pain and sciatica have been proven to respond better to natural movements than complete rest.[7]

The general approach to managing back pain emphasises a combination of activity, exercise and targeted therapies. Bed rest is typically only recommended for a short period, usually for no more than two days, and only for severe cases. Early movement, physical therapy, stretching, strengthening exercises and other non-invasive treatments are commonly prescribed to manage back pain and promote recovery. (As always, though, it's important that you get a diagnosis and that your therapist looks at your current lifestyle before making recommendations.)

Resting is not the best way to stop the pain.

Warming Up

The idea behind warming up is to gradually increase your level of exercise in order to prepare the body for what's about to come. This may be a light jog before sprints or some body-weight push-ups before heavy lifting in the gym. It's also good to work up a light sweat before you start to get yourself into the frame of mind for some exercise. However, the jury is out on whether it actually prevents injury.

When it comes to warming up before exercise, there are generally two types of stretching:

1. Static stretching: When you hold a single position for a period of time, such as bringing your leg back and holding it to stretch out your quad.
2. Dynamic stretching: When you take your muscles and joints through to their furthest movement, in a continuous motion.

Many studies have shown that warming up with static stretches has no impact on reducing the likelihood of injury and may actually be counterproductive.[8] The studies found that static stretching in top athletes:

- reduces strength in muscles by 5.5 per cent with a greater impact if the single stretch is held for 90 seconds or more (for less than 45 seconds the impact is minimal)
- reduces power in muscles by approximately 2 per cent
- reduces explosive power by a maximum of 2.8 per cent

Instead of static stretching, we know that dynamic stretching is better for your muscles and joints. You will have seen athletes and avid gym-goers warm up by doing movements that they are about to engage in. For example, football players swing their legs back and forth, and golfers practise their swing without the club in their hands. This is dynamic stretching and it has evidence behind it to show it helps with athletic performance and potentially the range of motion in joints.[9] Warming up with dynamic movement beforehand makes the motion less of a shock, and the muscles more able to handle the increased range required.

Though studies have shown that stretching has no significant effect on reducing muscle soreness after exercise or on reducing the risk of injury, in my personal opinion, stretching isn't going to cause you any harm.[10] I think putting your body through the motions of what you're about to do is a good thing for the mind–muscle connection. There is no harm in just getting your body, mind and muscles ready for the activity ahead.

If it feels good to stretch (and stretching can be quite individual in terms of how it feels, depending on age, past history with movement, duration, intensity and much more), then it is a great way to prepare yourself for exercise (pre-workout) or to end your workout (post-workout). Stretching in movement classes like Pilates and yoga can also be a great way to move your body and muscles.

If you're in pain and you keep feeling like you need to stretch, however, it may mean you need more than stretching to help reduce your discomfort, so please contact your healthcare provider.

REASONS TO WARM UP

I like warming up for three reasons:

1. Range of motion: Getting your joints slowly into full range of motion may help with depth or range when working out.
2. Focus: Some say that a warm-up mentally prepares you for the workout ahead. This may mean you focus better on form and indirectly reduce the chance of injury.
3. Body temperature: Dynamic warm-ups will increase your body temperature. This will get your blood pumping in your muscles, and it may help with endurance while working out.

What Exercise Is Best?

The majority of pain seems to be experienced when there is lack of movement, as inflammation builds up within the body if we stay still for a period of time. Our joints and muscles were created to move, so a lack of movement can cause stiffness and 'seizing up'. Some would argue that even just fidgeting in your chair is a great way to introduce some movement into your day.

When you exercise, it increases your heart rate, which causes vasodilation – an expansion of the capillaries within your muscles. This increase in oxygenated, nutrient-filled blood infuses into these areas to promote healing.

Many clients come to me asking what exercise they should do, but my answer is always the same: do whatever exercise works for you and that you enjoy doing! That will ensure you want to keep doing it and stay consistent, which is key when it comes to introducing a new exercise regime. If the exercise causes pain, discomfort, fear or anxiety, then it's unlikely that you will engage in it. Read through the different options below and decide what movement you could incorporate into your life that you will enjoy. Ask yourself:

1. What did you enjoy doing for exercise when you were younger?
2. How many times are you able to fit this movement into your week without it being a chore?

Once you've uncovered the exercise(s) that is right for you, take small, gradual steps to incorporate it into your everyday life (see page 103 for more guidance on this).

DON'T COMPARE

We now live in a world where people are showing how they are living their best lives on social media. It's easy to get sucked into believing that you need to be doing the same things and achieving the same stuff as others –

whether that's hitting the gym every day or doing 100 press-ups every morning. However, it's so important to note that you should not compare yourself to others who may enjoy types of exercise that you don't or may have been doing what you do enjoy for a lot longer. Remember, everyone started somewhere. It takes time and they've been exactly where you are now . . .

Exercise needs to be enjoyable for us to fit it into this busy life we all now lead.

LARA

Lara came to see me with lower back pain. She had seen another osteopath who had suggested that she needed to swim. However, after having three kids, Lara was lacking confidence in her body shape and therefore she didn't go swimming, nor did she do any other kind of movement as she thought that swimming was the only way she would solve her lower back problem. Her lower back pain became worse.

When I asked her, 'What movement would you like to do?', she said she would like to play badminton with her friends again, but she thought it was 'bad' for her back. I explained to her that all movement is good and as long as she doesn't jump in at too high an intensity, such as immediately entering a tournament, then her body will soon get used to badminton again. Like any new exercise, I told her to expect some soreness when she plays for the first time as it's a shock for the body, and not to be fearful of this.

Lara was really excited to be back playing badminton and glad she didn't have to get into swimwear at her local swimming pool. Within a few weeks, Lara was 80 per cent better and more open to other exercises like strength training (see below).

In terms of my favourite types of exercise that create the most benefit for muscles and joints, I would always favour loaded exercises, such as running or strength or resistance training. I also think swimming, Pilates and yoga are great as they use muscles and joints across different areas of the body.

Strength Training

People associate strength training with that intimidating corner of the gym, lifting weights and getting 'hench'. Women in particular often fear that they'll 'bulk up' or get too 'muscular' if they lift weights. However, when you lift weights, it burns body fat, and in order to get 'bulky' or more muscular you need to increase your calorie intake and change your diet to include much more protein. The truth is that strength training can be done within your limit at any age by using your own body weight. It has incredible benefits for your muscles and joints and doesn't even need to be done in a gym.

There are some exercises you can do that can help strengthen your back and body, and also encourage you to feel confident in the way that you move (see below). If you experience any persistent pain, it's worth seeing an osteopath to get a diagnosis and work together with them to strengthen your body.

THE FOUR BENEFITS OF STRENGTH TRAINING

1. Stronger bones: By increasing the load through our bodies, strength training can help with bone density, reducing the risk of osteoporosis and therefore pain.
2. Stronger joints: By building up the muscles around your joints, they can provide better support for your back.
3. Balance: I've found that when building muscle, my patients in clinic also have better control and balance skills, which reduces the chance of injury and therefore prevents pain from occurring.
4. Mental health: There's not enough research on this, but from those studies that have been done, there's evidence to show strength training can help ease symptoms of anxiety.[11]

So what is actually happening to your muscles when you strength or resistance train at home or in the gym? As I touched on in Chapter 1, when you stretch and contract your muscles it causes micro-tears in the muscle group. Your body then heals these micro-tears and fuses them together, creating a stronger and bigger muscle. This was shown in a study where participants trained one limb and not the other – there was a marked difference in the size of the untrained side compared to the trained side.[12]

Giving your muscles more strength can help to support your skeleton when performing daily tasks or sports. Daily tasks like lifting a box, vacuuming the house or carrying the grocery shopping will all be easier to do, and when I say sports this doesn't need to be playing football or golf every weekend – it can also just be playing with your kids in the garden or dancing round the kitchen. Strength training provides a better chance of not getting injured when doing these things.

The table below shows some key considerations when doing strength training:

Principle	Description
Warm up	Start with a warm-up to prepare your muscles.
Use the right weight	Choose an appropriate weight to maintain good form – proper technique is more important and has more impact than lifting heavier weights. Bear in mind this may mean going lighter than expected to begin with. Increase the weight gradually as your strength and form improve.
Maintain posture with bracing	Keep your back straight, engage your core (see page 97) and relax your shoulders.
Start with a solid base	Stand with your feet shoulder width apart and weight-balanced. Going barefoot is advisable because it helps you to balance more easily.
Breathe properly	Control your breathing: inhale before lifting and exhale during exertion.
Control the movement	Lift and lower weights with control, avoiding jerky movements.
Use full range of motion	Perform exercises through your complete range of motion, or lower the weight if it's too heavy.

Monitor your form	Pay attention to your form. Get feedback from others or record yourself and review the recordings. Ask a professional to help you with this if necessary.
Rest and recover	Allow proper rest between sets and workouts. Don't rush the workout.
Listen to your body	Stop if you feel pain or discomfort, and seek help if needed.

How you can strength train at home

- With one arm at a time, hold out a tin of baked beans in front of you with your arms straight for as long as you can and then hold it to the side of your body for as long as you can. Check that your neck is relaxed and your shoulders are soft away from your ears, without any tension. This is a great way to add weight to your arms and engage multiple muscles in your shoulders and elbows at the same time.
- Try doing press-ups gently against the kitchen worktop.
- While the kettle is boiling, do some wall sits to strengthen your glutes and legs. Stand with your back against a wall and your feet shoulder width apart, about half a metre away from the wall. Slide down the wall so that your knees are bent at a 90-degree angle and your thighs are parallel to the floor, or as far as you are able to go. Keep your back flat against the wall and your knees directly above your ankles. Hold this position, maintaining steady breathing for 15–30 seconds, gradually increasing the duration as you build strength.

- Perform some calf raises while you're waiting for the bus or train or for the kids to come out of school. Lift your heels off the floor, pause for a moment and then slowly lower your heels to the floor.
- While brushing your teeth, squat as low as you can go and then slowly push back up again.

These body-weight exercises will improve the strength and balance in your muscles and be beneficial for you.

MARVIN

Marvin, a 45-year-old male, came to see me with ongoing lower back pain after he had deadlifted a heavy weight in the gym. He was adamant that the deadlift caused this to happen and, in his words, 'broke his back'. He loved the gym as it was his way of clearing his mind and getting some alone time after busy days working as a lawyer in the City. However, he had come to terms with the fact that he wouldn't be able to go back again.

On examination, it was clear that Marvin had an imbalance in strength in his legs and glutes. He also seemed to have more muscle definition on the right side of his lower back.

I worked with him to give him specific exercises to help strengthen his back, while also encouraging him to go back to the gym, as he associated the gym with getting mental headspace from work. It was a shared decision about what he enjoyed doing in the gym and how we could implement those things around him doing some more specific rehabilitation for his back. In this case, I gave Marvin unilateral exercises (like lunges and single-leg glute bridges), which meant he was really able to focus on his weaker side.

Within two weeks, Marvin was out of discomfort and he was deadlifting again.

Swimming

Swimming is a great non-weight-bearing exercise that utilises lots of muscles and joints at the same time, and it has long been suggested as a way to help back pain. Breaststroke and butterfly involve arching your lower back, which may add some pressure to the lumbar vertebrae, while front crawl and back stroke maintain a low level of pressure throughout the body, so they may be easier to do if you have acute back pain.

Some people love swimming and swear by it, while others say that their back feels worse afterwards. The truth is that there is no way to tell whether you're a 'get better' swimmer or a 'get worse' swimmer until you try it.

What we do know is that swimming is a low-impact exercise that can help improve your overall fitness, flexibility and strength, which can all contribute to reducing the risk of back pain – and there are some pretty decent studies to show this also.

A systematic review and meta-analysis published in the *European Journal of Physical and Rehabilitation Medicine* analysed the results of eight randomised controlled trials and found that swimming was effective in reducing pain and improving functional ability in those with chronic lower back pain.[13]

But what if you hate swimming – because so many people do? That's fine! As I've said, you need to find something you enjoy, and there are so many other options that can help your back pain. There is no point in doing something you dislike.

Pilates and Yoga

Both Pilates and yoga are great, in my opinion, as they use body weight to gain movement through the joints. The slow, controlled movements and holding of the positions engages the muscles and allows for movement throughout your whole body. And, as we know, lack of movement is one of the main causes of pain. Cat-camel (see page 104), bridge pose (see page 100), downward dog and sphinx pose are all good yoga poses to ease back pain.

To go into downward dog:

- Begin on your hands and knees, with your wrists under your shoulders and your knees under your hips.
- Spread your fingers wide, press firmly into your hands and tuck your toes under. Lift your knees off the ground and straighten your legs as much as possible, forming an inverted 'V' shape with your body.
- Keep your head between your upper arms, with your ears in line with your upper arms and your back flat. Aim to press your heels towards the floor, even if they don't touch, so you feel a stretch through your calf muscles.

Sphinx pose is a gentle backbend.

- Lie on your stomach with your legs extended behind you, toes pointed and your elbows directly under your shoulders.

- Press your forearms into the ground and lift your chest up. Look forwards rather than up, keeping your pelvis and lower body on the floor.
- Your elbows should be shoulder width apart, your forearms parallel and your shoulders relaxed.
- Lengthen through your spine, gently drawing your shoulder blades down.

Many of my clients ask me which is 'best', Pilates or yoga, so here are the key points:

- Pilates improves posture, flexibility and overall muscle tone. It enhances body awareness, balance and coordination.
- Yoga increases flexibility, strength and balance. It reduces stress, promotes relaxation and improves mental clarity.

Remember, the best choice depends on your needs and preferences – find what brings you joy and keeps you healthy. Pilates is great for core strength, while yoga offers a balance of physical and mental well-being. But why limit yourself to just one when you can embrace both? Combining Pilates and yoga creates a well-rounded routine that suits your needs and keeps you motivated.

There are some preconceptions about Pilates and yoga. People assume that they need to be flexible to do them, or that they're not really 'proper' exercise. However, both Pilates and yoga are for all ages and abilities, and can definitely give your body an intense workout. There are always alternative exercises that are easier to do if you find a particular move more difficult. Both Pilates and yoga use strength and stretching, and can be done online or in person.

With both Pilates and yoga, you have to concentrate fully on the movements you are doing. With this in mind, you are also practising mindfulness and presence, which is a proven way to help reduce stress and therefore pain (as we'll see in the next chapter!).

Say hello to a more supple and agile you!

Running

When I see people in my clinic they often say they have a sore lower back, or sore hips and knees, and they will instantly blame the fact that they run, or even the fact that they used to run but have now given it up. In fact, there has long been a theory that running is 'bad' for you – that the weight going through your body is bad for your lower body, like your lower back, hips, knees and ankles, possibly predisposing you to arthritis. Now, I only run if I'm running towards an ice-cream van, so I can totally understand why someone would create this theory! However, it isn't true. Studies have found that runners' joints are actually really healthy. One study showed that runners had half the rate of osteoarthritis in their hips and knees compared to non-runners.[14] Another study has shown that we adapt our bodies according to the kind of surface we are on by adjusting the stiffness of our legs, and that we are well adapted for shock absorption.[15]

The reality is that running can help alleviate back pain by strengthening the core muscles and therefore better supporting your back. However, it's important to build up gradually and avoid high-impact activities until you have built up enough strength and stability. If you want to get started with running, as with other forms of exercise, it's important to begin with small steps. The NHS Couch to 5K app is a really good tool you can use for this (see Useful Resources, page 275).

There are also some ways in which you can put your body in an even stronger position to run:

- Strengthen your whole body: You don't just use your stamina and your legs when you run, you need to ensure your whole body is strong to maintain proper form.
- Hydrate: Keep drinking water, even when you aren't running.
- Footwear: Decent footwear can go a long way. Literally!
- Rest is OK: Be mindful of what your body needs. Check in with yourself and, when you feel rested, try to encourage some gentle movement again.

Go out and enjoy your runs!

Core Strength and Stability

Your 'core' refers to a group of muscles that work together to provide stability and support to your spine and pelvis. These muscles are located in your abdomen, back and pelvic region.

The core is an area of the body that people always talk about, but often it is misunderstood, so I am going to break down the anatomy of it so that you can visualise it and appreciate it for what it is:

- Rectus abdominis: This is the most well-known core muscle, commonly known as the 'six pack'. It runs vertically along the front of the abdomen and is responsible for flexing the spine (aka bending forwards).

- Transversus abdominis: This muscle lies deep within the abdomen and provides stability and support to the spine and pelvis. It is sometimes called the 'corset muscle' because it wraps around the midsection like a corset.
- Internal and external obliques: These muscles are located on the sides of the abdomen and are responsible for rotating and bending the spine.
- Multifidus: This muscle runs along the spine and helps to maintain spinal stability.
- Erector spinae: These muscles run along the length of the spine and are responsible for extending the spine (aka bending backwards) and maintaining the ability to stand up tall.
- Pelvic floor muscles: These muscles support the pelvic organs and are important for bladder and bowel control.
- Diaphragm: This muscle separates the chest cavity from the abdominal cavity and is important for breathing. It's often used in exercises like Pilates and yoga to help relax the muscles with effective breathing, helping the diaphragm function optimally.

The core is responsible for providing stability and support to your spine and pelvis, which helps maintain posture and balance. It acts like a natural corset, further protecting your spine from injury and reducing the risk of back pain. Strengthening your core provides better support for your whole body and back, enabling you to move more. Having strong core muscles can also improve athletic performance

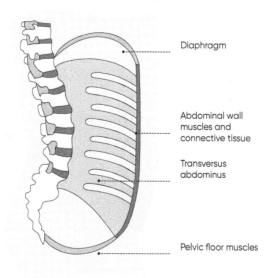

Diaphragm

Abdominal wall
muscles and
connective tissue

Transversus
abdominus

Pelvic floor muscles

and assist with breathing. By reducing the strain on your back muscles, the core muscles may help alleviate back pain and discomfort.

The evidence behind core exercises is mixed, like most evidence! However, if you start with the easier core exercises first and gradually build up, this will be a great way to see if your back responds positively to strengthening your core. Ideally, having some in-person sessions with a hands-on, experienced practitioner such as a Pilates teacher is the best way to make sure you are training with the best technique. I've included some core and stability exercises below for you and the plan on page 112 will guide you on how to incorporate these into your daily life. These four exercises should only take about five minutes to complete, so ideally try committing to doing these three times a week for eight weeks, to really make a difference to your back pain and core strength.

1. Plank:
   - Start in a push-up position with your arms straight.
   - Keep your body in a straight line from head to heels. Engage your core by bringing your belly button in.
   - Hold the position for 20–30 seconds, gradually increasing the time as you get stronger.

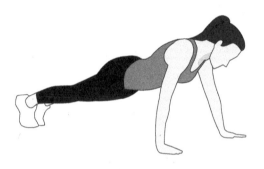

2. Bridge:
   - Lie on your back with your knees bent and feet flat on the floor.
   - Lift your hips towards the ceiling, forming a straight line from your shoulders to your knees.
   - Squeeze your glutes and hold the position for 20–30 seconds.

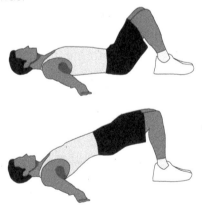

3. Bird-dog:
    - Start on your hands and knees in a table-top position.
    - Extend your right arm forwards and your left leg backwards, keeping your back straight.
    - Hold for a few seconds, then return to the starting position.
    - Repeat on the opposite side.

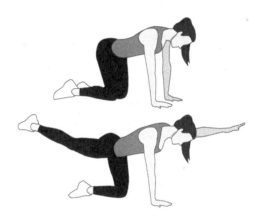

4. Dead bug:
    - Lie on your back with your arms extended towards the ceiling and your legs raised.

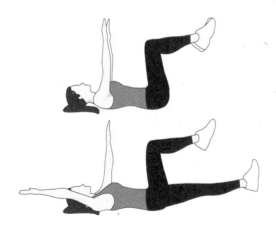

- Lower your right arm and left leg towards the ground without touching it, then hold for a few seconds.
- Return to the starting position and repeat on the opposite side.

OSTEO TOP TIP

Carry your shopping bags on one arm. Pull your belly button in but maintain slow, controlled breathing and walk to your car or home. This is a way to engage your core muscles in everyday life.

The above suggestions are some of the most popular ways to get movement into your day. However, I often see my clients trying to take on too much at once. If you're an all-or-nothing type of person, it's important to gradually increase your activity over a period of time, so that your body can adapt and not respond by giving you more pain – the weekly plan on page 112 will help you with this.

FRANCESCA

Francesca came to see me after struggling with pain for a long time. In her words, she had 'tried everything'. She was frustrated and angry and didn't feel like she should still be in pain at 35 years old. She was active and had heard that keeping moving was important, so she took that to a whole new level. She said that, on a weekly basis, she did yoga twice, Pilates once and strength training twice. She also walked 15,000 steps a day and her back

---

still hurt. I am not surprised she was angry with her pain! She was doing so much to try to solve it that it was probably exhausting her.

I looked at the list of things she was doing and asked her, 'Which one do you enjoy the most?' And she smiled and said, 'Well, I love strength training and yoga, and also I used to dance before this injury.'

So I told her to stop doing the stuff she didn't enjoy and explained that she was doing too much: 'A doctor doesn't give you ten pills for an ear infection. You get one and then if it doesn't work, you get another one.'

She did exactly this and found that she could move much more easily, and slowly but surely she was getting less pain in her back. This is a perfect example of how sometimes you can be doing too much for your body.

HOW TO BRING MOVEMENT INTO YOUR EVERYDAY LIFE

Sometimes we need a bit of advice as to what *actually* counts as movement. Below is what I tell my clients in clinic:

- Set yourself an alarm to get up from your desk and move at least every hour. There are also some good apps that can prompt you to do this.
- Try the simple routine below to mobilise your whole spine:
  - Thread the needle. Start on all fours in a table-top position. Extend your right arm fully under your body and twist your spine to reach to the left, as

far as you comfortably can. Your left hand can stay where it is, or you can extend your arm out in front of you for a deeper stretch. Hold this position and take deep, slow breaths for 20–30 seconds. You should feel a stretch in your upper back and shoulders. Repeat this on the other side.

o   Do a cat-camel stretch. Start on your hands and knees with a neutral spine. Slowly arch your back up like a stretching cat, then lower it down and let your stomach drop towards the floor, creating a sway in your lower back. Repeat this movement ten times.

- Walk to the kitchen to make a cup of tea.
- Walk up and down some stairs a few times.
- Take work calls while walking.
- Do laps of the house.
- Dance.
- Get outside for a walk or a jog.
- Do some gardening.
- Do the laundry.
- Lift some weights.
- Do a two-, five- or ten-minute simple mobility routine (see page 108).

These things can be done quickly and easily in short bursts.

Implementing Step 1: Keep Moving

I know it can be scary exercising when you're in a lot of pain. However, as you've now seen, this is actually one of the best ways to help reduce your pain. It's important, though, to take a gradual and cautious approach to getting back into exercise. Here are my top tips to help you do so safely:

- Consult with a healthcare professional: Before starting any exercise programme, it's important to consult with a healthcare professional such as a doctor, physiotherapist or chiropractor. They can help assess your injury and provide guidance on what exercises are safe and appropriate for you.
- Start with low-impact activities: Begin with low-impact exercises that don't put too much strain on your back, such as walking, swimming, cycling or gentle stretching.
- Focus on core-strengthening exercises: The muscles in your core help support your spine, so it's important to focus on strengthening these muscles.
- Incorporate stretching and flexibility exercises: Stretching and flexibility exercises, like yoga or Pilates, can help improve your range of motion and reduce muscle tension. Make sure you choose an instructor who is familiar working with clients with back injuries.
- Avoid high-impact activities while you're in pain: High-impact activities such as running or jumping can put strain on your back and increase the risk of re-injury. Avoid these activities until you have fully recovered and have built up enough strength and stability. You can gauge this by using the progress tracker on page 113. You should also notice a reduction in your symptoms.
- Listen to your body: Pay attention to how your body feels during and after exercise. If you experience pain or discomfort, stop the exercise and consult with your healthcare professional. It's important to progress slowly and avoid pushing yourself too hard, as this can increase the risk of re-injury.

> ### OSTEO TOP TIP
>
> Not all movements were created equal, but it's important to try to do what is within your means. If you are unable to do a full squat, do half a squat – that's fine. With time, you will be where you need to be. Just keep moving. Remember, progress is a beautiful process!

Movement can be just five minutes and it can really make a difference to your back pain and how you're feeling.

The importance of goal-setting when it comes to movement

It can be easy to set unrealistic goals for yourself when it comes to incorporating movement into your daily life, essentially setting yourself up for failure from the start. An example of an unrealistic goal is doing no training and then attempting to run the London Marathon. A more realistic goal is signing up for a parkrun (a 5km run) and gradually training for it using the Couch to 5K app (see Useful Resources, page 275).

Making goals realistic and conducive to your commitments and life is the key to engaging in movement and making a real difference to your pain levels and your mobility. One thing we know as healthcare professionals is that the outcome of treatment is better when there is shared decision-making or the individual is in charge.

Write down three movement goals that you'd like to achieve over the next eight weeks to a year, and then break them down into small steps so they are achievable. For example, if your goal is to go to the gym four times a week, consider how you can realistically fit this in once a week to begin with, and then build on that. Remember that what is realistic for you may be very different to what is realistic for other people, so try not to compare yourself. Regularly revisit your movement goals so you can see the progress you've made and whether there's anything you'd like to change. Writing down your goals and sticking them up somewhere visible – say, on the bathroom mirror or on your desk – can help to keep you motivated.

RYAN

Ryan came to see me with mid-back pain that was worse in the morning and at night. He works at his desk for eight to ten hours a day, runs his own company and has two kids.

Ryan mentioned that he wanted to set himself a goal of exercising for 30 minutes every single day. I worked with him to look at his busy schedule and set small targets. I explained that he should first give himself permission to do just 15 minutes of exercise a day. He could do this by playing with his kids in the garden at weekends and by stretching with them before bed. I showed how he could take work calls while walking outside, and he could get off public transport one stop early to walk or run to work if he wanted to.

When I saw Ryan four weeks later, he was smashing his daily 30-minute-a-day exercise goal and had lost 3kg. His mid-back pain had dissipated and he was more productive and energetic than ever.

In Ryan's case, we were able to incorporate movement into his lifestyle to make it work for him in a manageable way. Movement doesn't have to be long or hard work, but it can still make a big difference to your back pain.

OSTEO TOP TIP

If you operate from a paper or digital diary, it is really easy to slot in 5–10 minutes of movement throughout your day at regular intervals. This can be a short mobility routine at your desk or a walk away from your desk. Slot this stuff in as if it were an important meeting. If it's in your diary, then you're more likely to make time for it when you are super busy.

Simple mobility routines

If you're struggling to get started with incorporating movement into everyday life, try starting with the following two-minute mobility routine three times a week and gradually work your way up to the ten-minute version, perhaps four or five times a week. In time, this should give you more confidence with movement and enable you to commit to trying some of the other exercises outlined above.

Two-minute back pain mobility routine

1. Pelvic tilts: Lie on your back with your knees bent and your feet flat on the floor. Gently tilt your pelvis up and

back down, focusing on the movement in your lower back. Repeat ten times.

2. Knee-to-chest stretch: Lie on your back and bring one knee towards your chest. Hold for 15–30 seconds, then switch legs. Repeat once on each side.

3. Standing side bends: Stand up straight and bring your shoulder blades back. Let your hands rest on the side of your legs. Bend sideways at the waist as far as is comfortable and then go to the opposite side. Aim to do this at a slow and controlled speed (you are trying to get your joints/muscles moving).

Five-minute back pain mobility routine

1. Cat-camel stretch: See page 104.
2. Child's pose: See page 57.
3. Quadruped hip circles: Start on your hands and knees, and draw circles with your hips clockwise and counterclockwise. Perform five circles in each direction.

Ten-minute back pain mobility routine

1. Pelvic tilts: Same as the two-minute routine above.
2. Knee-to-chest stretch: Same as the two-minute routine above.
3. Cat-camel stretch: Same as the five-minute routine above.
4. Seated forward fold: Sit on the floor with your legs extended in front of you. Slowly bend forwards at the hips, reaching towards your toes. Hold for 30 seconds while maintaining a straight spine.
5. Bird-dog: See page 101. Perform ten repetitions on each side.

6. Hip flexor stretch: Kneel on one knee with the other foot planted in front of you. Gently push your hips forwards until you feel a stretch in the front of the back hip. Hold for 30 seconds, then switch sides.

Weekly plan

Below I've included an example plan for gradually increasing exercise. Remember, this is a bit like training a puppy to wee outside – you need to be consistent and not get too excitable if you want to ensure you're back to the gym feeling stronger than ever. Start by incorporating movement into your day at least three times a week, before gradually building up to 30 minutes of moderate-intensity exercise four or five times a week.

THE POWER OF HABIT STACKING

Something I often see in my clients is that they are given exercises by their physio or osteopath but they never remember to do them. If this is you, don't worry – it's super common and you're not alone.

Something you might find helpful when getting started on this first step is habit stacking: by combining your exercises with another activity that you do routinely throughout the day – such as having a cup of tea in the morning or a shower before bed – it can help to remind you to get them done.

For example:

Pain	Habit	Exercise
Central lower back pain	Brushing teeth	Wall sit (see page 91).
Sciatica back pain	Having a bath	Sciatic nerve flossing: also known as nerve gliding, this is an exercise designed to gently stretch and move your nerves to help them glide smoothly through the surrounding tissues. This can relieve pain and improve mobility, especially if you have nerve-related issues like sciatica or carpal tunnel syndrome. These movements often involve stretching and moving the limbs in specific ways to create a gentle pulling sensation along the nerve pathway, and I've seen my patients in clinic benefit a lot from doing them.
Mid-back pain	Washing up	Side bends (see page 109).
Dull ache – lower back pain	Getting to work	Park further away and walk.
Upper back pain	Watching TV	Seated cat-camel (see page 104).

Week 1: Establishing the foundations

- Start with 10–15 minutes of low-impact activities such as walking, swimming or cycling.
- Perform 2–3 sets of 8–10 reps of pelvic tilts, bridges and bird-dogs to begin strengthening your core.
- Incorporate gentle stretching exercises for your back muscles.

Weeks 2–3: Gradual progress

- Gradually increase the duration of your low-impact activities to 20–30 minutes.
- Continue performing 2–3 sets of 8–10 reps of pelvic tilts, bridges and bird-dogs to further strengthen your core.
- Incorporate a weekly yoga or Pilates class with an instructor who is experienced in working with clients with back injuries.
- Increase the duration and intensity of your stretching exercises.

Weeks 4–6: Consistent routine

- Increase the duration of your low-impact activities to 30–45 minutes.
- Add light resistance training with bands or light weights to your core strengthening exercises.
- Continue attending weekly yoga or Pilates classes, gradually increasing the intensity and duration of your practice.
- Increase the frequency and duration of your stretching exercises.

Weeks 7–8: Movement maestro

- Start incorporating some light jogging or jogging on a treadmill, gradually building up the duration and intensity.
- Continue with your resistance training for core strengthening.
- Attend yoga or Pilates classes at least twice a week, focusing on advanced poses that challenge your core strength and stability.
- Incorporate foam rolling or self-myofascial release exercises to improve your muscle mobility and reduce muscle tension.

Remember, this is just an example plan and it's important to consult with a healthcare professional to get personalised guidance based on your injury and fitness level.

When introducing movement into your life, especially when you have back pain, it's so important to give it time. I hope that by now, though, you've noticed a real difference in your pain levels. Continue to gauge your progress by filling in the tracker above every week and, remember, it's all about small steps and consistency.

'Keep moving' is the first step to healing your back. In the next chapter we will cover how changing your thinking might also be an important factor to consider.

PROGRESS TRACKER

Each week, rate the following statements based on your experiences using a scale of 1–5, where:

1 = strongly disagree

2 = disagree

3 = neutral

4 = agree

5 = strongly agree

- Pain intensity: My overall level of pain has decreased.
- Daily activities: Pain has impacted my ability to conduct my usual daily activities.
- Mobility and flexibility: I have noticed improvements in my mobility and flexibility.
- Exercise consistency: I have been consistent with my exercises and physical activity.
- Core strength: I feel stronger in my core muscles, supporting my back.
- Overall well-being: I feel more confident in my ability to manage and alleviate my back pain.

Filling in this progress tracker weekly can really help you to see how far you have come and the positive changes you have made.

Step 2: Reset Your Mind

IN THIS SECOND step we'll look at how you can reset your mind by becoming more aware of your stress response and the things that you are carrying that might be impacting your levels of pain. I'll dig into the science behind stress specifically, and give you tools to overcome your fight-or-flight response, adjust and refine your current mindset and subsequently help ease your back pain.

As with anything, our stress levels and the way in which we think are individual to us. Once you have read through the whole chapter, identify the areas that resonate most with you and try to implement at least one stress-busting strategy a week to reset your mind and take charge of your pain. Again, there is a weekly plan on page 146 to help you make gradual changes, and don't forget to fill in the progress tracker on page 148 to gauge how far you have come.

JENNY

I realised early on in my osteopathic career that there was more to back pain, or pain in general, than what people

---

feel. In fact, it happened in my first month of graduating from university.

There I was, a bright-eyed, bushy-tailed new graduate osteopath. I had my white coat on (mainly to ensure people didn't think I was a teenager) and I was loving my chosen path of 'fixing' patients with my bare hands. However, this was questioned when a patient called Jenny walked into my clinic room for the first time. When I took Jenny's medical case history, she talked about her back pain being excruciating and affecting her work deadlines. I asked how her stress levels were and she broke down in tears. Sobbing and reaching for a tissue, she said, 'To be honest, I'm going through a really nasty divorce at the moment as my husband cheated on me.'

I let Jenny talk and she then launched into details about her divorce proceedings and how she had found out about the affair. She also described how her parents were unsupportive of this decision and were trying to encourage the couple to work through it together. Jenny couldn't stop crying and all I could do was listen and offer her words of reassurance and support.

Once Jenny had told me her worries, I was almost out of time for the appointment and did an examination of her neck and upper back.

My shock came when Jenny jumped off the treatment couch and turned to me and said, 'Thank you so much. My goodness, my back feels so much better already.'

In that moment, I was confused. I knew stress and emotion could manifest in the body, but I had always had structural answers for this. For example, if you're worried or stressed, then your breathing changes and consequently it might cause rib pain. I had never seen pain diminish from someone just speaking with me.

I explained to Jenny that I hadn't actually treated her back in that first session, but that I thought she would benefit from seeing a therapist to discuss her personal life. She thanked me and also couldn't believe how connected her pain was to her current personal circumstances.

How could it be that in four years of university study we had not covered this in more detail? We had simply not gone into the complex realities of how pain manifests in the body. There have now been many studies that show how our brain is extremely clever at protecting us, but sometimes it needs to calm down a notch – and this chapter is going to teach you how to do just that.[1] As you read through the pages that follow, I want you to be open to looking at your emotional reactions and predictions for your pain, and be curious about how this might be impacting your pain experience and healing.

The Stress–Pain Cycle

Understanding the physiology of stress is so important when we're looking to take control of our pain, so let's start there. Your body is like a finely tuned machine, and the autonomic nervous system (ANS) is the control system that keeps everything running smoothly without you consciously thinking about it. It's like the computer in charge of your body's functions, such as heart rate, blood pressure and breathing. The ANS has two main branches: the sympathetic and parasympathetic systems.

The sympathetic system is like your body's accelerator pedal. When you face stress or danger, it jumps into gear, triggering what is commonly known as the 'fight-or-flight' response. Stress can affect all of us in different ways. Sometimes you don't even know you're stressed, but you wake up and realise you've been clenching your jaw all night, or that you have been breathing differently. Some forms of stress are acute and sudden like a panic attack, while others are slow builders. Many of my clients report an increase in their pain levels when they are going through a tough time at work or in life.

On the other hand, we have the parasympathetic system, which is like your body's braking system. It helps you calm down after the stressor is gone, slowing your heart rate, promoting things like digestion and allowing you to relax and recover. This is often referred to as the 'rest and digest' response.

Together, when working in harmony, these two branches of the ANS keep your body in balance, responding to various situations as needed. Let's look at this more closely now.

The acute stress response

Acute stress refers to a short-term and immediate response to a perceived threat or challenge. It is a normal and temporary reaction that occurs when we encounter demanding or threatening situations. Acute stress can be triggered by various factors, such as work pressures, exams, public speaking, conflicts or unexpected events.

When faced with acute stress, the body activates the 'fight-or-flight' response, leading to the release of stress hormones like adrenaline and cortisol. Physiologically, acute stress can manifest as increased heart rate, elevated blood pressure, rapid breathing, heightened alertness and tensed muscles. These changes prepare the body to respond to the immediate challenge, enabling quick decision-making, enhanced focus and increased physical capabilities. These reactions are a survival mechanism that allows us to fight off or flee life-threatening situations.

Let's look at what this acute stress response might look like in real life.

Say you feel a sharp pain in your back after lifting a sofa. In the first stage of the acute stress response, the amygdala part of our brain (which deals with emotion) signals the brain stem to release epinephrine and norepinephrine (aka adrenaline and noradrenaline). Once released into the blood, these will increase your heart rate, breathing rate and blood pressure and make you have more visible reactions like sweating and dilation of your pupils. Importantly, this short sympathetic response promotes inflammation to eliminate foreign invaders or pathogens (see page 23).

Approximately 15 minutes after the onset of stress, cortisol levels increase across the whole body, helping to mobilise energy resources and heighten focus and alertness. These levels remain elevated for several hours.

This acute response is beneficial in short-term stressful situations. For example, a temporary stress reaction to pain, or even non-pain-related stress, may provide us with important information that will protect us from further harm (for example, not attempting to lift the sofa again).

However, when the body is in chronic – long-term – stress, this can mean that we get 'stuck' in a stress–pain cycle, where stress causes pain and pain causes stress.

The chronic stress response

In the case of a chronic long-term stress response, such as ongoing back pain when you wake up every single morning in agony, prolonged exam preparation or ongoing stressful life circumstances, cortisol secretion can become consistently elevated. This can have a profound negative impact on your physical and psychological health – for example, leading to an increase in inflammation, and therefore aggravating your back pain, or causing you to limit your quality of life from fear of it becoming worse.

Cortisol is produced by the adrenal cortex (a part of your kidney that is key to the stress response). Throughout the course of your day, cortisol serves to protect your body against harm by maintaining blood glucose levels and giving more energy to the busy brain and nerves, by putting less energy into underused body parts. For example, it will give more energy to your digestive system while you are eating and to your muscles while you are running for the bus. Cortisol is also a powerful anti-inflammatory hormone; it can prevent and reduce the inflammation caused by injured muscle tissue and nerve damage.

Despite its important role in the body's daily function, the ongoing and consistent release of cortisol when the body is under chronic stress – a bit like a constantly leaking tap – can actually do the reverse and increase inflammation in your body by disrupting the hormone signals from the brain, which obviously isn't great news, especially when it comes to pain. An increase in inflammation can lead to feeling more pain in our joints and muscles. Some studies have even reported that non-pain-related stressors can trigger the amygdala in the brain and create pain even if there is no damage within the body.[2]

It has been shown that if stress is pain-related – for example, bending over to take the washing out of the washing machine and feeling a sharp pain in your back – then cortisol can actually exacerbate the experience of this pain and, furthermore, it may even create a fear-based memory of this pain.[3] This leads to a hypersensitive physiological stress response. Imagine your body's pain alarm system being overly sensitive, like a smoke detector that goes off at the slightest whiff of smoke, even when there's no real fire. So, when someone with a hypersensitive physiological stress response experiences pain, their body tends to react strongly, as if there is a significant danger or threat.

Our bodies are amazing and they are trying to protect us. Studies have demonstrated, though, that our cortisol levels rise in anticipation of a stressful event and the amount varies according to our brain's decision about how important this threat is.[4] Putting more emphasis on pain will therefore make your pain worse.

This sort of fear-based stress response and focus on pain increases cortisol secretion and then makes the pain worse.

These repeated stressful reactions in our body can lead to, and eventually cause, cortisol dysfunction. As we've seen, cortisol is our body's natural anti-inflammatory. It is amazing, but when it isn't working properly, it causes complications such as conditions like rheumatoid arthritis, fibromyalgia, chronic fatigue syndrome, temporomandibular (jaw/ear/temple) joint pain, ongoing lower back pain, sciatica and more. Without cortisol functioning and monitoring inflammation levels, our bodies end up having no control over stressors that are pain- or non-pain-related.

Inflammation leads to cell and systemic tissue damage, and the signs and symptoms of stress-induced cortisol

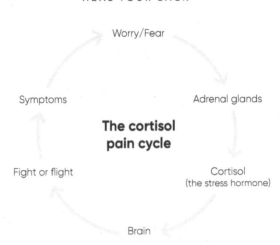

Worry/Fear

Symptoms

Adrenal glands

**The cortisol
pain cycle**

Fight or flight

Cortisol
(the stress hormone)

Brain

dysfunction are possible fatigue, depression, bone and muscle breakdown, pain, trouble with memory and more.[5] Like with many things, it's all about balance – we need just the right amount of cortisol. If we compare it to food, for example, it's like putting just the right amount of balsamic vinegar on the salad, otherwise Gordon Ramsay is going to send it back! Too much will overpower the mozzarella and too little will result in no taste at all.

The Psychological Effects of Stress and Pain

Being in a constant state of heightened awareness and stress can also lead to ongoing, recurrent negative thoughts or worry. Our thoughts and our beliefs have a huge but invisible impact on everything in our lives, and particularly in terms of how we deal with or approach pain. Perhaps you believe that you have a 'weak' back because your dad has always had back pain and people say you 'have your dad's body'. Or maybe you believe that there is always going to be danger when you walk out of the door as you once got mugged and it was a traumatic experience for you.

Often patients come to see me with the narrative of 'My posture is so bad' or 'Back pain runs in my family so it was bound to happen.' We all have internal narratives or stories that we tell ourselves about pain – maybe yours is playing out in your head right now. These narratives can be about how much pain we expect to feel, how long it will last or what it means for us. These stories can actually have an impact on how our bodies respond to pain.

Research has found that the way we think and talk about pain can influence our actual experience of it.[6] The more we engage in negative thinking around our pain, the more likely we are to keep doing so in the future, which can further compound the pain. This negative thinking – or negative pain narrative – can often lead to catastrophising, which in turn will prolong the release of cortisol. As we've seen, this can really take its toll on our body, both physically and psychologically. 'Catastrophising' is when our thoughts lead us down a path of feeling like the worst thing is going to happen. Of course, this can happen in everyday life – like being late for work and thinking that you're going to be fired – or indeed for pain.

Pain catastrophising is described as the tendency to magnify the intensity of pain and to feel unable to deal with the pain stimulus. It is also the inability to reduce pain-related thoughts before, during or even after the painful event has taken place. An example of catastrophising when it comes to back pain might be a thought process like, 'I have had pain in my back for a few days; it may mean that I will be like this forever and I may need an operation.'

These beliefs may result in an exaggerated stress response

that, as we saw above, is proven to increase and prolong the pain experience.[7] More importantly, what I see in clinic is that pain is a standalone stressor in its own right. Therefore, it can exacerbate this stress response in the brain and contribute to chronic pain. The pain itself causes stress, but then we worry about what that pain means, asking ourselves questions like, 'What happened?', 'Why do I feel this way?', 'What does this mean now and for my future?', which then exacerbates the stress response – it's that vicious circle again. Is this something that resonates with you? If so, there are some gradual steps below to help you break free of this cycle and reset your mind.

HOW STRESS MIGHT IMPACT YOUR BODY PHYSICALLY

The stress response is a physical release of chemicals in the brain that in turn cause a bodily reaction. Acute stress might occur in the form of a panic attack or being sick, and chronic stress can lead to ongoing back pain or irritable bowel syndrome (IBS). In clinic, I've noticed that, when there is anxiety or stress, it can affect people in many ways:

- Breathing: If you're anxious or having a panic attack, you will notice that your heart rate might change and then your breathing also changes. This can affect the muscles between your ribcage, called the intercostal muscles. The nerve supply to your diaphragm is also from the top of your neck, so all of this can cause aches and pains from your neck down to your mid-back.

STEP 2: RESET YOUR MIND

- Sleep: Sleep is so important that it's a step in itself (see Chapter 6), but here is a tiny snippet. Anxiety and stress can disrupt your sleep in a big way. Have you ever found yourself lying awake at night agonising over a project or worrying about a family member? Sleep is so important for us in more ways than we realise and especially when it comes to helping our body to heal itself.
- Gut health: There is strong evidence to suggest that stress can play an important role in gut health.[8] Alongside the sympathetic and parasympathetic nervous systems, there is a third branch – the enteric nervous system. This is sometimes referred to as the 'second brain' as it involves lots of nerves within the walls of our digestive system. The enteric nervous system plays a crucial role in maintaining our gut and controlling the release of digestive enzymes to help break down our food. These three branches mediate the brain–gut connection and any alterations in this can play a role in why IBS symptoms occur.

How to Control the Stress Response

It can be difficult to break free of this stress–pain cycle, but I want to reassure you that it is possible to do so – now we'll explore how.

Stress is considered a natural part of daily life and occurs in varying amounts. It may not be practical to try to live in a world free of stress. However, there are several ways in which you can calm down your nervous system, release any underlying stresses and therefore reduce your pain. Read through this section and try to introduce at least one tool a week and see if it makes a difference to your pain levels. There is also a weekly plan on page 146 that will guide you in making gradual mindset changes.

Mindfulness

One way of calming down the sympathetic nervous system and therefore moderating our pain is through being able to become more present – through mindfulness or meditation, for example. These practices involve focusing the mind on the present moment and observing thoughts, emotions and bodily sensations without judgement. They can help us to step out of our brain, look at a situation and decide whether it is dangerous or not. The goal is to cultivate a non-reactive awareness of our pain, and to develop a more accepting attitude towards it. Being more present in the moment allows us to stop focusing on and worrying about our pain.

Below are my top three tips to being more mindful:

1. Concentrate on breathing in for a count of seven and out for a count of seven.
2. Focus on your five senses and ask yourself: 'What can I feel, what can I see, what can I hear, what can I smell, what can I taste?'
3. Concentrate on something you can see in front of you or pick it up. Look at it carefully and try to describe it in your head. Although this may only take a few minutes, it's highly effective at bringing your mind into the present.

These methods distract your mind from the stress you are experiencing and enable you to become more present in the moment, which means you are able to calm down and relax more. Mindfulness has amazing benefits for you, and research has shown time and time again that it can hugely impact your mind and body.[9] Try one of these methods now and see if it helps you to relax.

Visualisation

Visualisation is imagining a positive scenario to help distract your mind from your negative thought patterns. This can be a bit like meditation in some ways, but instead you are closing your eyes and maybe imagining a positive outcome to what you are currently experiencing. Try the following exercise:

- Close your eyes and take a few deep breaths to relax.
- Visualise yourself in a peaceful and serene environment, such as a tranquil garden or a quiet beach.
- Imagine a warm, healing white light surrounding your body, sinking into the areas of pain and discomfort.
- With each inhale, envision this light bringing relief and comfort to those areas.
- As you exhale, imagine releasing any tension or negativity stored in your body.

Visualisation could also take the form of imagining yourself being really strong in the gym and lifting heavy weights without being in pain.

Deep breathing

Have you ever noticed how, when you experience pain, your breathing changes? And when you are scared or stressed your breathing becomes faster paced and shallower? When we experience pain or even fear of pain occurring, our heart rate may go up. This is our brain predicting or feeling pain or discomfort. Taking slow, deep breaths helps the heart rate to go down. When you breathe deeply, you are allowing more oxygen to enter your body and you are expanding your ribcage. Your heart rate also increases slightly and, as you breathe out, your heart rate slows. Slowing your breath down is a way of getting your heart rate to match your breath. This is why so many meditation techniques focus on slow and deep breathing.

Breathing deeply stimulates the vagus nerve, which is the main nerve of the parasympathetic system. Stimulating the vagus nerve promotes relaxation by slowing down your heart rate. This reduction in stress and anxiety will also change the way in which your brain then perceives pain. Anatomically, deep breathing creates better movement through your ribs and this in turn will help increase mobility through your mid-back and diaphragm. And, as we know, better mobility and movement leads to a decrease in pain.

Give this a try now:

- Put your hands on your stomach and slowly take a deep breath in through your nose to fill your chest; feel your hands on your stomach rise up. Do this for a count of ten seconds.
- Now slowly let the air come out of your lungs and let your hands drop back down for a count of ten seconds.
- Repeat this five times.

Deep breathing is a great stress-reduction tool and can be done every single day as a way of relaxing. You're breathing *anyway*, so you might as well make the most of its amazing powers. Perhaps do the above breathing technique before you go to sleep every night, or after you've had breakfast. It is also very effective to do this when you're actually experiencing pain.

I often tell my patients when they wake up in the morning with pain to take five deep breaths into their tummy. This slows their heart rate down and allows their muscles to relax before they get out of bed. This reduces stress and over time reduces the likelihood of waking up in pain, in a positive cycle. Again, everyone responds differently: I've had people respond straight away and feel calmer and more relaxed, and others take a week to feel the benefits of deep breathing.

Altered focus

Close your eyes, think of another part of your body that isn't painful and imagine it slowly warming up to a comforting temperature, such as in a warm bath. Focus on that body part feeling warm and notice how your pain levels reduce slightly. This is another way of distracting yourself from the back pain that you are experiencing. This can be an effective mechanism to distract from and therefore reduce the stress associated with the pain, and reduce cortisol levels.

Mindful walking

Mindful walking is a great way to bring relaxation into your life, as being in nature is automatically calming. When you are walking, notice how your feet feel when they touch the ground and what the breeze feels like on your face. Listen to the birds and maybe cars around you, but be present and aware of your senses in this moment. Just 10–15 minutes of mindful walking is enough time to calm the stress response.

Social support

We must also talk about the importance of having a social support system. Research shows that having a support system in the form of friends or family can help to reduce your stress levels.[10] When you have a strong support network, you become more resilient to stress and experience fewer stress symptoms like increased heart rate or broken sleep patterns. If you are feeling overwhelmed or stressed, try reaching out to a close friend or family member this week to offload or just hang out with. I know that, personally, this always helps to reduce my stress levels.

Time out

Taking time out doesn't have to mean spending lots of money and going somewhere hot; just being outside in the natural light and relaxing at home meditating can also be considered a break for your mind and body. This is an amazing way of helping your cells, muscles and bones recover – as well as giving your mind a rest from the stresses of everyday life. I can't tell you how often my patients come in to see me in clinic and say they had zero back pain while on holiday!

Do a body scan

This technique involves systematically directing attention to different parts of the body and observing bodily sensations without judgement. This can help to relax the body, release tension and stress held in the body and therefore reduce pain.

Find a comfortable and quiet space to sit or lie down. Close your eyes and take a few deep breaths to relax.

1. Start with your toes: Bring your awareness to your toes. Notice any sensations or tension. Take a deep breath in and, as you exhale, imagine releasing any tension in your toes.
2. Move to your feet: Slowly shift your focus to the soles of your feet. Feel the connection with the ground. Inhale deeply and, as you exhale, let go of any tightness or discomfort in your feet.
3. Shift to your ankles and calves: Gradually move your attention upwards, scanning your ankles and calves. Breathe in and, with each exhale, release any tension stored in this area.
4. Focus on your knees and thighs: Continue the scan, directing your awareness to your knees and thighs. Inhale deeply and, as you exhale, allow any stiffness to dissolve.
5. Move to your hips and pelvis: Bring your attention to your hips and pelvis. Feel the support beneath you. Take a deep breath and, as you exhale, let go of any tightness in this area.
6. Scan your lower back: Gently shift your focus to your lower back. Inhale, imagining fresh air filling this space and, as you exhale, release any tension or discomfort.
7. Proceed to your upper back and shoulders: Move up to your upper back and shoulders. Inhale deeply and, with each exhale, release the weight and tension you may be carrying in this area.

8. Focus on your arms and hands: Direct your awareness to your arms and hands. Inhale, feeling the energy in your limbs, and exhale, letting go of any tightness or stress.

9. Scan your neck: Gradually move your attention to your neck. Inhale deeply and, as you exhale, release any stiffness or tightness in this area.

10. End with your head and face: Finally, bring your awareness to your head and face. Inhale and, with each exhale, let go of any tension in your jaw, forehead and scalp.

Open your eyes and take a moment to observe how your body feels. This simple body scan technique, when practised regularly (at least three times a week, but ideally more), can enhance relaxation and reduce pain by promoting mindfulness and releasing stored tension in your muscles as you breathe and relax each body part.

OSTEO TOP TIPS

Below are my top tips for reducing stress and cortisol levels.

- Go for a five-minute walk.
- Put on an upbeat song and dance around for the duration of the music.
- Write down ten times: 'My body is fierce and strong.' I've found that this has helped my patients feel less fearful and more positive about their pain.

Reconnect with things you enjoy

You can even shift to things that your brain used to enjoy as a way of gaining some insight and clarity into your pain. By shifting your brain and thoughts to a positive time and experience, you may be able to rewire and replicate how you felt in that moment. In the same way that the negative narrative reinforces negativity, a positive narrative can help to activate the parasympathetic nervous system. One of my patients, who was in her seventies and an ex-professional musician, had to stop playing her violin due to her mid-back pain. The inability to play had caused her stress and was possibly contributing to her pain response. I suggested that she reconnect with her music by listening to her favourite violin concerto when she was at home. This made her feel more positive and able to respond more favourably to the exercises and treatment I was giving her. Is there anything you can reconnect with this week that brings you joy?

Change your mindset

In recent years, neuroscientists have found that our mindset can also influence our perception of pain.[11] There are many types of mindset, but the main ones I want to focus on here are:

- Growth mindset: A growth mindset is the belief that your abilities, intelligence and talents can be developed and improved through dedication, effort and learning from mistakes. If you have a growth mindset, you see challenges as opportunities for growth, embrace failures as stepping stones to success and are motivated to learn and continuously improve.

- Fixed mindset: A fixed mindset is the belief that your abilities, intelligence and talents are fixed traits and cannot be significantly changed. If you have a fixed mindset, you tend to avoid challenges, fear failure and criticism, and may believe that your abilities are predetermined. You often focus on proving your existing skills rather than developing new ones.

- Negative mindset: A negative mindset refers to a generally pessimistic and defeatist outlook on your life and circumstances. If you have a negative mindset, you often perceive difficulties as insurmountable obstacles, dwell on problems rather than seeking solutions and expect negative outcomes. This mindset can hinder personal growth, create a cycle of negative thinking and limit opportunities for success. It is understandable that suffering with pain in the long term can lead us to become more susceptible to this negative thought pattern. In my experience, the key is to become aware of these thoughts so that you can then change them.

- Positive mindset: A positive mindset is characterised by an optimistic and constructive approach to life and challenges. If you have a positive mindset, you tend to focus on possibilities, solutions and opportunities. You believe in your ability to overcome obstacles, learn from setbacks and find positive aspects even in difficult situations. A positive mindset can foster resilience, motivation and personal growth.

You might recognise yourself in some of the descriptions above. Perhaps you think 'I know I am stuck with back pain forever now' or 'No doubt I'm going to need surgery on this back soon, otherwise I might not be able to walk in a few years' time.' These are examples of fixed and negative mindsets.

DON'T FEAR PAIN

When you've been in agonising pain for years it's hard to imagine a life without it. As we've seen, pain is complex – it's multifactorial, which means that there are many things that can impact it. This can include your thoughts around pain. Pain doesn't always reflect the amount of damage. For example, paper cuts are very painful but only small. With guidance, you can work on your perception of pain and feel more confident about the strength of your body.

I have included a mindset questionnaire below to help you identify your dominant mindset around your pain. Remember, mindset is not fixed and can be changed over time with awareness and intentional effort. Use this questionnaire as a starting point for self-reflection and then read on to find out easy tips for changing this.

PAIN MINDSET QUESTIONNAIRE

Please read each statement below and select the response that most closely aligns with your thoughts and behaviours. There are no right or wrong answers; this questionnaire is designed to help you identify your mindset tendencies when it comes to pain. Be honest with yourself and answer based on your genuine reactions to pain and challenges.

---

1. When faced with physical pain:
   a. I see it as an opportunity for personal growth and resilience.
   b. I view it as a setback and an indication that something is wrong with me.
   c. I feel overwhelmed and defeated, assuming the worst will happen.
   d. I try to stay positive and focus on the lessons pain can teach me.

2. In the face of a persistent challenge or chronic pain:
   a. I believe that my efforts and perseverance can lead to improvement.
   b. I tend to think that the situation will never get better, no matter what I do.
   c. I feel stuck and helpless, thinking that nothing can change.
   d. I search for ways to adapt and cope with the ongoing challenge positively.

3. When discussing pain with others:
   a. I'm open to sharing my experiences and learning from theirs.
   b. I prefer to keep my pain private, fearing judgement or pity.
   c. I often complain about my pain, expressing negativity and hopelessness.
   d. I focus on finding solutions and supporting others in similar situations.

4. **Reflecting on past experiences of overcoming pain or challenges:**
   a. I see them as valuable learning opportunities that shaped who I am today.
   b. I tend to remember the negative aspects and feel a sense of victimhood.
   c. I feel resentment and frustration, dwelling on the unfairness of the situation.
   d. I appreciate the strength and resilience I demonstrated during those times.

5. **When encountering setbacks or worsening pain:**
   a. I view them as temporary obstacles that can be overcome with effort and learning.
   b. I see them as proof that I'm not capable of handling challenges.
   c. I become disheartened and question my ability to cope with life's difficulties.
   d. I focus on finding alternative strategies and solutions to address the setbacks.

Scoring:
   ☐ Count the number of times you selected a, b, c or d.

Interpreting your results:
   ☐ Mostly a and d: You likely have a growth or positive mindset, emphasising learning, resilience and adaptation in the face of pain or stress.

□ Mostly b and c: You may have a fixed or negative mindset, tending towards feelings of helplessness, victimhood or a negative outlook.

It's always valuable to reflect on your limiting beliefs and actively work towards cultivating a more growth-oriented and positive mindset. As an osteopath working with people in chronic pain, I see time and time again how a negative mindset around pain has an impact on how well my clients respond to treatment and also their willingness to take simple steps to relieve their pain. In addition, as we've seen, if we constantly tell ourselves that our pain will be unbearable or long-lasting, our bodies may respond by intensifying the pain sensations. The longer these pain narratives stay the same, the more they become ingrained. However, you have the ability to change your mindset and these internal narratives – and that is down to something called neuroplasticity (I love this word so much that I actually debated calling my dog Neuroplasticity – Neuro for short).

THE POWER OF NEUROPLASTICITY

For a long time, it was widely believed that the brain and its processes were relatively fixed and unchangeable. This belief stemmed from the idea that the brain reached its full development during childhood and adolescence, after which it entered a state of stability with limited capacity for change. This perspective suggested that our cognitive abilities, behaviours and even our thoughts were fixed.

However, over the past few decades, ground-breaking discoveries in neuroscience have revolutionised our understanding of the brain's capabilities. The concept of neuroplasticity emerged, challenging the long-held belief in the brain's static nature.

Neuroplasticity refers to the brain's remarkable ability to change and reorganise itself throughout our lives as a result of learning and experience. Which is good news when it comes to negative thinking around pain. Our brains are changing all the time – and we have a choice about where to direct them.

You have a choice about how to change your brain,
by where you focus your thoughts.

Our brains have the ability to change at their own pace, and that creates hope when it comes to helping your back pain and being able to improve at doing almost anything you want to. It is this combination of strength and confidence that really makes an impact on how our brains perceive back pain and therefore how we react to it. This is the exciting part! Research has shown that, if we have a more positive or optimistic outlook, our bodies may respond with less intensity or discomfort.[12] When we are stuck in a fixed mindset about our pain, we become trapped in negativity and our neural pathways work against us. However, when we learn to adopt a growth mindset, the opposite happens and we can 'unlearn' our pain.

Below are the tools that I give my patients to help to change their mindset around pain and also help them to control their pain. I really hope they enable you, too, to embrace a mindset of 'I will get stronger and learn how to manage my back pain' or 'I'm going to be totally fine and I know this is all normal.' Try incorporating one of these tools daily each week and see what impact it has on your pain.

Change your pain narrative

By becoming aware of our thoughts and the stories we tell ourselves about pain, we can actively work on modifying them. This means we can shift from negative or fearful narratives to more positive and empowering ones – and, as a result, reduce our pain.

Changing our internal narratives doesn't mean ignoring or denying the reality of pain. It means acknowledging the pain, but focusing on resilience, coping strategies and the potential for improvement. By doing so, we can actually influence how our bodies perceive and process pain, leading to a more manageable and less distressing experience.

To start, you will find below a copy of a pain catastrophising scale.[13] This scale is designed to provide you with a quantitative measure of your tendency to engage in catastrophic thinking about pain. I'd like you to spend a few minutes answering these questions:

1. **How often do you find yourself imagining the worst possible outcome when you experience pain or discomfort?**

- 0: not at all
- 1: rarely
- 2: occasionally
- 3: frequently
- 4: all the time

2. **When you are in pain, do you feel helpless or overwhelmed, believing that nothing can be done to improve your discomfort?**

- 0: not at all
- 1: rarely
- 2: occasionally
- 3: frequently
- 4: all the time

3. **Do you magnify the significance of your pain, perceiving it as much worse than it is?**

- 0: not at all
- 1: rarely
- 2: occasionally
- 3: frequently
- 4: all the time

Now add up the numbers to get your total score. The closer you are to 12, the more likely you may be catastrophising your pain.

If this exercise revealed that you have a tendency to catastrophise when it comes to pain, there is an easy way to change your narrative.

A pain management tool I use with my patients in clinic aims to reframe their pain mindset. It has powerful results, so I want to share it with you. Telling yourself that pain is 'bad' or that you are 'broken' is telling yourself that this is how you will be. However, changing the words you use can help your recovery. Grab a journal or notebook and a pen. Think about your pain and write down how you feel about it and what your fears are around your pain. Pick out the negative narratives and reframe them – for example:

Instead of . . .	Try . . .
I am broken.	I am sore but I am strong.
I can't lift this, it hurts.	This feels sore right now.
I am going to be in pain forever.	My body takes time to heal.
Pain runs in my family.	Pain isn't hereditary.
I have a bad back.	Sometimes I get a sore back.
I hate my body – it keeps falling apart.	I am grateful for my body and for being alive.
I got injured so I can't do my gym workout.	Once I got injured in the gym but I'm fine now.

Try to do this exercise daily. However, if that seems overwhelming, then start by doing it three times a week and committing to certain days when you can do this. You'll soon see a difference in how you think about your pain.

KABIR

Kabir, a 42-year-old man, sought my help with a history of persistent back pain. Having consulted with multiple specialists without finding lasting relief, he expressed feelings of despair and self-doubt. His narrative not only consisted of physical symptoms, but also negative

---

thoughts about his own body and capabilities. He kept saying he was 'broken' and that his 'body and his back were a nightmare case'.

I recognised the connection between Kabir's back pain and his mental state. I made sure I listened to him and acknowledged how frustrating it must feel to have seen multiple specialists and not to have had an improvement. I explained how I didn't think he was broken and that actually I believed we needed to reframe his belief system. He agreed to commit to trying to reframe this.

I introduced Kabir to the concept of cognitive reframing. We systematically identified negative thoughts and beliefs he held about himself and his body during my hands-on treatment sessions. Through dialogue and reflection, we replaced these thoughts with positive, empowering words and affirmations.

Together we created the mantra, 'I am feeling sore at the moment, but my body is strong.' This became a part of Kabir's daily routine. He also then used this affirmation in moments of back pain, gradually reshaping his internal dialogue.

Over a few weeks, Kabir reported a noticeable reduction in the frequency and intensity of his back pain. Equally, there was a positive shift in his mindset and confidence in his back.

Encouraged by his progress, Kabir gradually reintegrated into activities he had avoided due to his condition. Playing with his son in the garden and doing light workouts at the gym became parts of his routine, contributing to a huge shift in his confidence and outlook.

After a few months, Kabir, armed with a newfound confidence and positive narrative, decided to participate in a local 10km run for charity.

Through a personalised approach that combined cognitive reframing and positive affirmations, Kabir not only found back pain relief, but experienced a profound shift in his self-perception.

Affirmations

An affirmation is a positive statement aimed at encouraging a desired mindset or outcome. It's a tool commonly used in mindfulness and self-help to reframe your thoughts and beliefs. When it comes to back pain relief, affirmations can be used as a way to complement other tools to reduce discomfort and promote a more positive mindset. Examples of affirmations for pain relief include statements like 'I am capable of managing my pain' and 'With each breath, I release tension and invite relaxation into my back.' These sorts of affirmations can help you shift your focus away from pain sensations and bring a more positive, empowered perspective to your back pain.

Give your pain a name

Therapists sometimes ask people to name their anxiety so that they can detach themselves from it. I often encourage my clients to do the same with their pain. Give your pain a name . . . like Sally (this is not intended as a negative to any Sally who may be reading this). This will enable you to detach yourself from the thoughts that you are having and also to treat it like something you can show compassion and empathy towards. Remind Sally (your pain) that you are strong and you are OK. For example, try saying, 'Sally, don't be so annoying – my body is strong.' I know this sounds a bit 'out there', but believe me, it really does work when it comes to changing your pain narrative! What name could you give to your pain?

Accept your pain

Accept that pain happens to everyone and you are not to be blamed for any of it. Most of us instantly want to blame something or someone to help us better understand what is happening. But the truth is that pain is normal; it is a part of life. Pain is like having a cold – we don't always know who gave it to us (unless you have children who go to nursery); we just accept that we have a cold and our body is having to fight it. We also know that, with time and the right tools, a cold will go away again. This is the same as back pain – it is extremely common and it is likely that you will have days of discomfort and they will vary in degrees of pain. Try to reassure yourself that, even though it's inconvenient or you feel a bit rubbish, it will pass, especially when you use the tools in this book.

Don't compare your pain to others'

Not everyone has the same pain threshold or the same injury. Your lower back pain might feel worse compared to someone else's for many reasons, so do not compare your recovery journey to someone else's. This is often hard as we live in a world of social media and it is easy to compare these things, just like body image. Remember, no two bodies are the same! If you are struggling with comparison, try taking a break from social media or reducing the time you spend on it each day, and curate your feed by unfollowing those accounts that bring up negative feelings for you.

> *If you can change your thinking, you can change your pain.*

Implementing Step 2: Reset Your Mind

When you're in pain, it's normal to feel extra stress about it. Below are a few quick wins you can try to help reduce your stress before moving on to the weekly plan.

- Digital detox: Designate specific times for a digital detox – for example, limiting screen time in the evenings.
- Quality sleep: Prioritise quality sleep by maintaining a consistent sleep schedule and creating a calming bedtime routine.
- Gratitude practice: Daily, jot down three things you're grateful for. Reflect on positivity to shift your focus.
- Self-care rituals: Introduce a daily self-care ritual like a warm bath, reading or listening to calming music.

Weekly plan

Week 1: Establishing the foundations

- Daily deep breathing: Start with five minutes of deep breathing each morning. Focus on your breath, inhaling deeply through your nose and exhaling through your mouth.

- Give your pain a name: Try the technique on page 144 and see if it helps to distance you from your pain.
- Physical activity: Incorporate ten minutes of light stretching or a short walk into your daily routine.

Weeks 2–3: Introducing relaxation techniques

- Continue with your daily deep breathing and add in a body scan before bedtime.
- Mindful walks: Extend your daily walks to 15–20 minutes. Practise mindful awareness of your surroundings.
- Positive affirmations: Repeat positive affirmations to yourself in the morning and before bed.

Weeks 4–6: Building mindfulness practices

- Mindfulness: Introduce a daily mindfulness session for 10–15 minutes. Explore the different mindfulness techniques on page 126, or try progressive muscle relaxation or loving-kindness meditation, which involves focusing on generating and sending out positive emotions through a series of structured steps. The goal is to increase your compassion and empathy, which can improve your emotional well-being and relationships with others. There are several guided progressive muscle relaxation and loving-kindness meditation exercises online.
- Take time out: Take a look at your diary and see if you can schedule some time out – even if it's just for a few minutes – this week.

- Social media: Check in on your social media use and set limits or curate your feed if you feel it is affecting your stress levels.

Weeks 7–8: Consolidation and advanced techniques

- Reframe your negative pain narrative: Begin keeping a stress journal. Write down your fears about your pain and reframe them.
- Social support: Engage in regular conversations with friends or family. Share your stress reduction journey and seek support.
- Advanced mindfulness practices: Attend a mindfulness class or use advanced guided meditations. Practise mindfulness in daily activities, such as when eating or commuting.

The simple tools you have introduced in this step will enable you to break free from the stress–pain cycle and change your thinking around pain. Keep going with your daily practice and remember to track your progress to see how far you have come – you will really start to notice a difference in your pain levels.

Now, let's delve into the next step, which explores how nutrition and eating habits can impact and alleviate back pain. This section will provide you with manageable and quick ways in which to implement nutritional changes into your daily life.

PROGRESS TRACKER

Remember to fill this in weekly, rating the following statements based on your experiences using a scale of 1–5, where:

1 = strongly disagree

2 = disagree

3 = neutral

4 = agree

5 = strongly agree

- Pain intensity: My overall level of pain has decreased.
- Daily activities: Pain has impacted my ability to conduct my usual daily activities.
- Mobility and flexibility: I have noticed improvements in my mobility and flexibility.
- Exercise consistency: I have been consistent with my exercises and physical activity.
- Core strength: I feel stronger in my core muscles, supporting my back.
- Stress levels: I feel more relaxed and less stressed.
- Mindset and attitude: I have noticed positive changes in my mindset and attitude towards managing my back pain.
- Overall well-being: I feel more confident in my ability to manage and alleviate my back pain.

CHAPTER 5

Step 3: Eat Well

ALTHOUGH I AM not a dietician or a nutritionist, during many years of working as an osteopath I have seen how eating the 'right' sort of food can not only have a positive effect on your health, it can also impact the way in which the body interprets pain. A lot of my clients come to me with general pain, not specific to any muscles or joints, or they notice an increase in their pain after eating specific foods. Often, this is a sign of potential inflammation within the body. In these circumstances, I refer them to a nutritionist who gives them some core tools to manage their pain through diet. These are the tools I will share with you in this step.

In this chapter, I'll walk you through the ways in which you can make small changes to your diet to help your level of pain. This is not a quick fix, but it's worth looking at what you consume and whether it might be causing or contributing to your pain. After all, we *are* what we eat.

Once again, this step is all about making small, gradual changes. There is a weekly plan to support you with this on page 184, and don't forget to fill in the progress tracker on page 186 so you can monitor any positive impact on your pain levels.

Following an Anti-Inflammatory Diet

Inflammation is often the focus when looking at how nutrition impacts pain. As we saw in Part 1, inflammation is both good and bad for us. Inflammation is our body's immune response to infection and viruses, and it is what kicks our body into action to help get rid of those annoying illnesses. However, chronic inflammation can lead to multiple issues, including back pain. It's therefore worth considering whether your diet is contributing to inflammation – and therefore exacerbating the pain in your body.

Some foods that can trigger inflammation include:

- refined carbohydrates, such as white flour and white rice
- fried or processed foods (see below)
- processed meats, such as ham and sausages
- sugary food and drinks, including fizzy drinks
- alcohol

These are known as proinflammatory foods. A lot of research has shown that diets that restrict these proinflammatory foods and introduce those that are anti-inflammatory can help to reduce back pain.[1]

Anti-inflammatory foods

Below are some specific foods that have anti-inflammatory properties:

1. Fatty fish: Fatty fish, such as salmon, mackerel and sardines, are rich in omega-3 fatty acids, which have

been shown to have anti-inflammatory properties. Studies have suggested that consuming omega-3 fatty acids may help to reduce inflammation in the body and may benefit those with conditions such as rheumatoid arthritis, asthma and inflammatory bowel disease (IBD).[2] Including polyunsaturated fatty acids and omega-3 within our diets has been proven to be beneficial for osteoarthritis.[3] Omega-3 fatty acids and vitamin B12 also provide support for nerve-related pain like chronic back pain with sciatic involvement.

2. Berries: Berries, such as blueberries, raspberries and strawberries, are rich in antioxidants. Studies have suggested that consuming berries may help to fight free radicals and reduce inflammation in the body.[4]

3. Leafy green vegetables: Leafy green vegetables, such as kale, spinach and cabbage, are rich in nutrients such as vitamins C and E, which have been shown to have anti-inflammatory properties.

4. Nuts: Nuts, such as almonds, walnuts and pecans, are rich in healthy fats and antioxidants, and may help to reduce inflammation in the body.

5. Turmeric: Turmeric is a spice that contains a compound called curcumin. Studies have suggested that consuming turmeric or curcumin supplements may help to reduce inflammation in the body and may benefit people with conditions such as arthritis.[5]

While the evidence supporting the anti-inflammatory properties of these foods is not yet conclusive, incorporating these foods into a balanced and varied diet may help with reducing inflammation in the body – and therefore reducing pain.

PROCESSED FOOD

Processed food refers to food items that have undergone various alterations from their natural state, such as drying, canning, freezing or adding preservatives, flavourings or other chemicals. Below are some characteristics of processed foods:

- Additives: Processed foods often contain additives such as preservatives, artificial flavours, colours and sweeteners to enhance taste and appearance and increase shelf life.
- Texture modification: Processing can alter the texture of foods, making them tastier or more convenient for us to eat. This includes things like grinding and milling, which are techniques commonly used in the production of snack bars, cereals and processed meats.
- Increased shelf life: Preservation methods such as canning, freezing and vacuum packaging extend the shelf life of processed foods, allowing them to be stored for longer periods without spoiling.
- Convenience: Processed foods are often convenient and ready to eat or require minimal preparation, appealing to those seeking quick meal solutions in today's fast-paced world.
- Higher salt, sugar and fat content: Many processed foods contain high levels of salt, sugar and unhealthy fats to improve taste, which can contribute to health issues such as obesity, cardiovascular disease and diabetes when consumed in excessive amounts.
- Lower fibre content: Fibre is super important for digestive health, as you'll come to see, but processing can remove or reduce the fibre content of foods.

Examples of processed foods include canned vegetables, packaged snacks, frozen meals, breakfast cereals, deli meats and prepackaged sauces and condiments. While not all processed foods are unhealthy, nutritionists advise consuming them in moderation and choosing options with minimal additives and nutrient loss.

Ultra-processed food

Ultra-processed foods are those that have undergone multiple changes that take them away from their natural state. As an example, plain cornflakes are a processed food; however, adding sugar, colourings or artificial flavourings make them ultra-processed.

Now, I am not advocating that you follow a 'strict' diet; incorporating more anti-inflammatory foods doesn't have to be hard work or mean making big changes to your everyday diet. Ultimately, an anti-inflammatory diet is simply one that many nutritionists refer to as a 'balanced' diet, so let's now take a quick look at the different components of a balanced diet and how they may impact inflammation, your muscle and joint health, and your pain.

Carbs, protein and fat: What you need to know

Carbohydrates, protein and fat are known as macronutrients and are the nutrients found in food that give you energy and keep your body functioning.

Carbohydrates

Carbohydrates often get a bad rap, with many people advocating a low-carb diet, but they are an important energy source. They are stored in the liver and muscles as glycogen and are then used as and when the body exerts itself and needs this energy for physical activity.

Not all carbs are created equal, though. Refined carbohydrates, such as white bread, pastries, biscuits and pizza, might aggravate inflammation, which, as we've seen, can exacerbate pain in the body. Wholegrain carbohydrates, such as brown rice or pasta, oats, quinoa, wholegrain breakfast cereals and wholewheat bread, may therefore be a better choice and have the added benefits of containing a range of vitamins and minerals, including folate, calcium, iron and B vitamins.

Protein

Proteins are long chains of amino acids, which are the building blocks in your body, sort of like Lego pieces that come together to form something epic. These proteins have vital roles, such as helping your muscles grow, fixing injuries and serving as 'workers' for various tasks in the body. Amino acids act like kitchen helpers for enzymes, ensuring that chemical reactions in your stomach run smoothly. They even play a role in supporting your immune system, hormone production and energy backup supply. I think of them as one of the key ingredients to keep your body feeling its best and working as a finely tuned machine!

It's important to consume protein at each mealtime. Current protein recommendations are 0.75g per kilogram of body weight a day in adults. However, if you are very active, then the guidelines suggest that you could eat more than this per day.

The best sources of protein are lean meats like chicken, turkey and pork, as well as fish and eggs. However, vegans and vegetarians can also get protein from foods such as tofu, lentils, quinoa, nuts and seeds. It's important for both vegans and vegetarians to consume a variety of these foodstuffs to ensure they are getting enough essential amino acids. Although things like protein shakes are beneficial if you are in a rush, they are ultra-processed (see box above) and don't provide for all your body's needs like food can.

Fats

Fat is often demonised, with supermarket shelves bulging with low-fat options. However, these often contain additives and other 'fillers' that make them far from healthy. Fat is important in our diet as it helps with the absorption of some vitamins like vitamin A, but it is also a super concentrated source of energy and fatty acids that are needed for growth and health. There are different forms of fats and these play a part in inflammation and how it may aggravate back pain.[6] Our individual gut microbiome will also play a role in how our bodies respond to fat, but more on gut health later (see page 167).[7]

High-quality omega-3 fatty acids – found in flaxseed oil, chia seeds and oily fish like salmon – have been shown to have anti-inflammatory properties.[8] Introducing these foods into your diet can help to reduce the levels of inflammation in your body. Processed and fried foods, on the other hand, contain omega-6 fatty acids, which have been shown to have proinflammatory effects.[9] Interestingly, quite often I find that my patients have a healthy diet that contains lots of oily fish and healthy oils, but they also contain high levels of omega-6 in some shape or form. This means that the omega-3 they are consuming isn't having the desired anti-inflammatory effect.

THE IMPACT OF BODY WEIGHT ON PAIN

A number of studies have shown that a higher body mass index can contribute to adding pressure on your spine and joints (hip and knee joints), and consequently lead to pain.[10] Obesity and weight gain can also lead to inflammation in the body, thereby exacerbating or even leading to chronic pain. Eating a balanced diet can help you to keep to a healthy weight and will have a positive impact on your pain. It's also worth looking back at Chapter 3 and seeing what small steps you can implement when it comes to movement. I know it can seem daunting, but gradual steps are a good way to get started. If you lack confidence in the strength of your body, take a look back at Chapter 1 and remind yourself that our bodies and our spines are strong. The mindset tools in Chapter 4 may also help you to reframe your thinking.

Fruit and vegetables

When the body is in an inflammatory response, it produces unstable atoms known as free radicals. These are a vital part of our body's reaction to help us fight infections. However, they can also have an impact on our healthy cells and this may lead to something called oxidative stress. Oxidative stress is a form of inflammation and can lead to muscle and spine pain and stiffness, as well as a feeling of achiness in parts of the body. Fruits and vegetables are rich in micronutrients, such as vitamins A, C and E, as well as antioxidants, which can help to defend healthy cells from being wrongly attacked by these free radicals.

However, when chronic inflammation is present, our antioxidants may be depleted and so we get into a vicious cycle where inflammation introduces more free radicals, which in turn cause further inflammation. Eating a healthy, balanced diet with at least five portions of fruit and vegetables a day or a variety of 30 different plant foods a week can help to break this cycle and reduce your pain.

Below is a checklist you can use to keep track of what you already include in your weekly selection of fruits and vegetables, and also to give you a few more ideas about what you can introduce into your weekly menu.

Fruit and vegetable checklist

Fruits

o	apple	o	fig
o	apricot	o	grapefruit
o	avocado	o	grapes
o	banana	o	kiwi
o	berries (blackberries, blueberries, raspberries, strawberries)	o	mango
		o	melon
		o	orange
		o	papaya
o	cherries	o	passionfruit
o	coconut	o	peach
o	cranberries	o	pear

o   pineapple   o   tangerine
o   plum   o   watermelon

Vegetables

o   asparagus   o   leek
o   aubergine   o   mushroom
o   beetroot   o   onion
o   broccoli   o   peas
o   brussels sprouts   o   pepper (green, red,
o   carrot   yellow)
o   cauliflower   o   potato
o   celery   o   radish
o   courgette   o   spinach
o   cucumber   o   spring greens
o   garlic   o   sweetcorn
o   green beans   o   sweet potato
o   kale   o   tomato

Something I'm hearing more about in clinic is 'Type B' malnutrition. Jessica O'Dwyer, a clinical nutritionist who I regularly recommend to my clients, told me: 'This form of malnutrition is characterised by a calorie-rich but nutrient-poor diet, making individuals susceptible to chronic, low-grade infections and, in turn, chronic inflammation. A diet balanced in essential nutrients can tackle this issue effectively.'

WHAT DOES A BALANCED DIET LOOK LIKE?[11]

According to the UK government's Eatwell Guide, we should aim to eat at least five portions of different fruit

---

and vegetables a day, and they should make up just over a third of the food we eat each day.

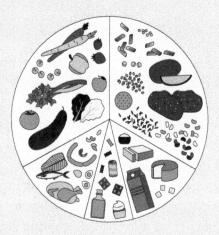

Starchy food, carbohydrates such as bread, potatoes, rice and pasta, should also make up just over a third of the food we eat. Where possible, we should choose higher-fibre or wholegrain varieties.

We should also be eating some beans, pulses, fish, eggs, meat and other protein foods. It's best to choose lean cuts of meat, and eat less red and processed meat like bacon, ham and sausages. When it comes to fish, we should aim for at least two portions (2 x 140g) of fish every week, one of which should be oily, such as salmon, sardines or mackerel.

A balanced diet also includes some dairy or dairy alternatives (such as soya drinks and yoghurts). Milk, cheese and yoghurt are good sources of protein and are an important source of calcium, which helps keep our bones healthy.

When using oil and spreads, we should choose unsaturated options and eat them in small amounts.

Foods that are high in fat, salt and sugar, such as chocolate, cakes, biscuits, sugary soft drinks, butter, ghee and ice cream, should be eaten less often and in small amounts.

As we'll come on to below, drinking 6–8 cups or glasses of water a day is also important. Lower-fat milks, lower-sugar or sugar-free drinks and herbal teas all count towards your daily intake.

As you can see, we need a good balance of all these things for our bodies to lead epic lives. A diet that contains more processed foods and is lacking in essential nutrients can lead to inflammation and cause pain and discomfort in our backs. Your diet is the fuel that you give yourself for energy and it should be varied, balanced and bring you joy.

MARIA

Maria is 35 years old and used to run regularly, but stopped going out much and exercising due to family issues at home. She had been hit by a car when she was 28 years old and it had left her with some ongoing intermittent lower back pain. She came in to see me because she felt 'unfit' and like her body was 'getting old'.

On questioning Maria, I realised that her diet had changed considerably since she'd had some family difficulties and had started a new, demanding job in the city. She mentioned that her diet mainly consisted of quick meals like instant noodles or baked beans on toast. When I asked Maria about fruit, vegetables and wholegrains, she said she didn't eat much.

I asked Maria to include two portions of oily fish in her diet a week and to try to eat three different types of vegetables a day – this could include pulses. I also asked her to take vitamin D every day and supplement her diet with turmeric in her cooking or curcumin tablets.

Within about four weeks, Maria reported a marked difference in her range of movement and her general feeling of health and well-being.

Maria is a great example of how diet can impact the way your body feels. Even if you make some small changes initially, they can have a big impact further down the line. Time is often a limiting factor when it comes to having a balanced diet. Where necessary, you can always take supplements to help support your nutrition.

WHAT ABOUT INTERMITTENT FASTING?

Intermittent fasting (IF) has become a bit of a trend in recent years, with fans claiming it can improve everything from weight loss to brain function. But did you know it could also potentially help alleviate pain in our bodies? Let's dive into the evidence . . .

First, let's define IF. It's a pattern of eating where you alternate periods of fasting (abstaining from food) with periods of eating. There are different ways to do it, but the most common methods include the 16:8 method (fasting for 16 hours and eating within an eight-hour window) or the 5:2 method (eating normally for five days and restricting calories to 500–600 for two non-consecutive days).

So, how can IF help with pain? Well, studies have shown that it can decrease the levels of inflammatory markers in the body, which can potentially reduce pain.[12] But wait, there's more! IF has also been shown to increase the production of endorphins, the body's natural painkillers. Endorphins are released during exercise, laughter and even when eating chocolate (yes, really!). So, by fasting, you're potentially increasing the production of these feel-good hormones, which can help alleviate pain.[13]

Of course, as with any diet or lifestyle change, it's important to consult with a healthcare professional before starting IF, especially if you have any underlying health conditions. And let's be real, fasting can be challenging at times. But the good news is that you can still enjoy your favourite foods within your eating window, which means you don't have to give them up entirely.

So, while more research is needed, the evidence suggests that IF could potentially help alleviate pain in our bodies.

Supplements That Help with Back Pain

Supplements may be prescribed by doctors or musculoskeletal therapists to aid their patients on their journey to reduce pain and discomfort.

There are a *lot* of supplements, so consequently not all of them have adequate studies to fully show their benefits when it comes to pain. However, below are those that do show some evidence of working:

Fish oil (omega-3)

Actual fish is always going to be better for you than the pill version. However, supplements that include oils or fatty acids, such as argan oil,[14] olive oil capsules rich in polyphenols[15] and fish oils that are rich in omega-3, have been linked to a significant reduction in pain in people who have osteoarthritis.[16,17,18] There have also been studies on exercise-induced pain, researching the effects of supplementation with omega-3 derived from fish oil, and these found a significant reduction in musculoskeletal pain after consumption.[19,20,21]

Recommended dosage: 3,000mg per day for an adult.[22] The NHS recommends two servings of fish a week, of which one should be an oily fish like salmon.[23]

When it comes to back pain, calcium, vitamin D and magnesium are important too:

Calcium

Calcium is known for helping to support bone density, but it also helps with the absorption of vitamin D. Calcium can be obtained from dairy and leafy green vegetables like broccoli and kale. It helps with the formation of bones, which can reinforce our backs and help them to continue to be the strong structure that they are designed to be.

Recommended dosage: 700mg per day.

Vitamin D

Sunshine – that's what I think of every time someone says vitamin D to me! It is such an important vitamin as it helps to regulate calcium and phosphate in the body. This helps to keep our muscles, teeth and bones healthy. Studies have shown that vitamin D also helps to reduce pain in those who have chronic pain.[24]

Though vitamin D is found in some foods, such as oily fish, red meat, liver, egg yolks and fortified foods, it's difficult to get enough vitamin D from food alone.[25] From March to September, we should all get enough vitamin D from sunlight, but it's important to consider supplementation during the autumn and winter months if you live in the northern hemisphere.

Recommended dosage: 10–20mg per day.

Magnesium

Magnesium is an essential mineral that supports nerve and muscle function in the body. It works together with calcium and vitamin D to maintain strong and healthy bones, aids in calcium absorption and plays a role in bone formation and density. Magnesium is also essential for proper muscle function, including muscle contraction and relaxation. It helps to prevent muscle cramps, spasms and soreness. There is some suggestion that it helps with chronic pain.[26] Magnesium is also a mineral that can help you sleep better, which is so important when it comes to pain felt in your body (see Chapter 6 for more on this). Foods rich in magnesium include nuts, spinach and wholemeal bread, though a supplement can also be taken.

Recommended dosage: 300mg for men and 270mg for women per day.

Creatine

Strangely, this is the most researched of all supplements and it's also the one that isn't as widely publicised by healthcare professionals or in the media for its benefits. Most of the research has been centred around the fact that it helps with recovery from exercise, and might consequently have other health benefits including less pain.[27] It is the most popular supplement among personal trainers as it has been shown to fight muscle fatigue and help with power output. This is super beneficial in those who lift weights intensely, which I appreciate isn't everyone,[28] but some studies have shown that it also appears to reduce mental fatigue in mentally demanding scenarios and sleep deprivation.[29,30] This may help when dealing with stress and deadlines, which, as we saw in the last chapter, can also contribute to – or even cause – pain.

Recommended dosage: 3–5g per day or 0.1g per kg of body mass per day. To be taken before or after exercise.[31]

Curcumin

Curcumin, or turmeric, has been used for many years in cooking within certain cultures. I can definitely remember my mum grating fresh turmeric and squeezing the juice from it, mixing it with ginger and lemon and giving it to me when I had a cold or flu as a child. So you can imagine her shock when she saw all the turmeric shots and juices on the shelves of our most well-known supermarkets. She still to this day claims she did it first and could have been a millionaire! But does it actually work? Well, yes! There is some promising evidence that it can help with some types of pain as it works as an anti-inflammatory. The main studies conducted seem to be centred around knee osteoarthritis; however, the results are promising.[32]

Recommended dosage: 1g per day.[33]

Collagen

Collagen is a protein that forms part of the structure of various connective tissues in the body, including bones, tendons, ligaments and cartilage. The intervertebral discs, which act as shock absorbers between the vertebrae, contain collagen. As people age, the collagen content in these discs may decrease, contributing to conditions like degenerative disc disease and back pain. Although the research is limited, the idea behind using collagen for back pain is that it may help support the health of the discs in the spine and the surrounding connective tissues.

Recommended dosage: 5–15g per day.

The Role of the Gut Microbiome

Our guts are made up of trillions of micro-organisms, including bacteria, fungi and viruses, known as the gut microbiome. Everyone's microbiome is individual to the person and can be influenced by many things including the first food you ate as a baby,[34] your stress levels,[35] if you've taken certain medications, especially antibiotics,[36] and even where you live![37]

These micro-organisms are both helpful and potentially harmful for the body. The 'good' bacteria help break down food and absorb nutrients, and also protect us from 'bad' bacteria. When there is a healthy balance of bacteria in the gut, it's called symbiosis.

The more variation in your gut microbiome, the healthier the gut.

However, when there is an imbalance – known as gut dysbiosis – it can trigger systemic inflammation. When the gut is inflamed, it can lead to a condition called leaky gut syndrome. Jessica O'Dwyer says, 'When the gut membrane is compromised – a condition known as "leaky gut" – unwanted substances can leak into the bloodstream, triggering an immune response and, consequently, systemic inflammation. This inflammation is a critical link between gut health and pain, including back pain.

'The cycle of inflammation originating from a compromised gut barrier can set off a cascade of events that sensitise pain receptors throughout the body. This means that a compromised gut membrane can exacerbate existing pain or even initiate new pain experiences, such as musculoskeletal discomfort or back pain. Restoring gut membrane integrity can break this cycle. It involves removing irritants and allergens from the diet, repairing the gut lining with specific amino acids like L-glutamine, and rebalancing the gut microbiota with beneficial bacteria through the use of probiotics (which contain live beneficial bacteria) and prebiotics (which feed the beneficial bacteria in your gut). By comprehensively addressing gut health in this way, we not only alleviate digestive issues, but can also make significant strides in reducing inflammation and, by extension, pain.'

The gut microbiome also has a big role to play in how we feel. There has been an abundance of research to show a connection between our gut and our mental health. Evidence shows that 90 per cent of serotonin is produced in our gut, and not only does it help to break down our food, it also helps with our emotions.[38]

Why is this important to pain? Well, serotonin is our feel-good hormone – it helps us sleep better, feel less stressed and have better mood. If there is an imbalance in our serotonin, this can impact how we feel and this in turn won't help our mindset when it comes to managing our pain.

People who have IBD conditions like ulcerative colitis or Crohn's disease often experience changes in their gut microbiome. However, there is now new evidence to show that a change in your gut microbiome may also lead to other painful conditions like fibromyalgia, headaches, inflammatory pain, other chronic pain conditions and even painkiller tolerance.[39] With this in mind, it makes sense for those of us suffering with back pain to take steps to maintain our gut health. If we can help to balance the good and bad bacteria in our gut, we can not only reduce inflammation, but also increase our levels of serotonin and improve our mood, which all contributes to reducing pain.

Jessica O'Dwyer says, 'Poor diets that are low in fibre and high in saturated fats and sugar are often culprits for gut dysbiosis', so again it comes down to trying to eat a balanced diet as much as possible. Try mixing up the kinds of vegetables and fruit you're eating regularly. Be daring and try something new this week!

Below are some practical steps you can take to balance your gut:

1. Incorporate fibre-rich foods: Aim for a diverse range of fruits, vegetables, wholegrains, legumes and nuts. These foods are high in fibre, which serves as a prebiotic.
2. Include fermented foods: Integrate fermented foods like yoghurt, kefir, sauerkraut, kimchi and miso into your diet. These foods are probiotic and can help replenish and maintain healthy gut flora.
3. Choose polyphenol-rich foods: Polyphenols are plant compounds found in foods like berries, green tea, dark chocolate and olive oil. They have antioxidant properties.
4. Consider a probiotic supplement: If you're not getting enough probiotics from food, consider taking a high-quality probiotic supplement. Look for a product that contains a variety of strains, including *Lactobacillus* and *Bifidobacterium*.
5. Include prebiotic-rich foods: Foods rich in prebiotics include garlic, onions, leeks, asparagus and bananas. These compounds nourish the beneficial bacteria in your gut and help them stay happy and thrive.
6. Stay hydrated: Drinking enough water supports overall digestive health and helps maintain a favourable environment for your gut bacteria.

Food Intolerances and Back Pain

Food can impact how we feel and how we heal, so it's important to think about what it gives us in terms of nutrients, as well as how you feel after you eat certain foods – sometimes they may leave you feeling bloated or uncomfortable compared to other foods.

Food intolerances are becoming increasingly common, mainly because we now have more access to a variety of different foods, which can sometimes have an impact on our gut. Food intolerances are caused by the body's inability to digest certain types of food properly. This can be due to a lack of digestive enzymes or other factors that prevent the body from breaking down the food properly. As a result, the food stays in the digestive system for longer than it should, causing irritation and inflammation in the gut.

Many people experience symptoms such as bloating, wind, diarrhoea and stomach pain after eating certain foods. However, food intolerances can also cause other symptoms, including back pain and muscle aches and pains. Our reactions to food tell us something and it's important to take note of this and make the changes required to help reduce our back pain.

The reason why food intolerances can cause back pain and muscle aches and pains is that inflammation can affect the entire body. When the immune system is activated, it releases inflammatory chemicals that can cause pain and discomfort in the muscles and joints. In addition, when the gut is inflamed, it can lead to malabsorption of nutrients, which can contribute to muscle weakness and fatigue.

Some common foods that can cause intolerances include gluten, dairy, soya and eggs. If you're experiencing these types of symptoms and suspect that you may have a food intolerance, it's worth considering the role that food intolerances may be playing in the pain that you are experiencing. By identifying and eliminating problem foods, you may be able to improve your overall health and well-being and, most importantly, the pesky back or joint aches and pains. However, it's important to speak to your healthcare professional before eliminating anything from your diet. There are many amazing nutritionists and functional medicine doctors who can help with this.

OTHER GUT CONDITIONS ASSOCIATED WITH BACK PAIN

- IBS: IBS is a diagnosis that is given to many people who experience unexplained stomach symptoms. These can range from abdominal discomfort or cramps, to intermittent constipation and then diarrhoea. It is estimated that between 68 and 81 per cent of people with back pain will experience IBS.[40] The cause of this hasn't been properly researched, but it is believed to be due to referred pain from the stomach to the back, as the muscles tighten to compensate. Inflammation within the gut may cause this referral pain. In clinic, I've had patients who have reported lower back and mid-back pain when they've had an IBS flare-up.
- Constipation: Constipation causes inflammation within the digestive tract, and studies have shown that it can cause referred pain in the lower back, lower limbs and whole body.[41] However, there need to be more clinical trials in this area to further determine whether there is a direct link.
- Bloating and wind: This is usually just uncomfortable and a minor annoyance. However, there is also a connection between these symptoms and back pain. There's no concrete reason, but it is thought that

when the bloating and wind are intense, it might cause referred pain in the back.

- Acid reflux: Acid reflux results in burning in the oesophagus and abdominal pain. This can also result in referred pain in the mid-back or lower back in some patients.
- Crohn's disease: Lower back pain is reported in 52 per cent of those with Crohn's disease.[42] Most commonly it is due to axial arthritis, which involves pain and stiffness across the lower back and sacroiliac joints. Crohn's not only impacts your stomach, it can also impact other areas. It is good to look at your lifestyle and treat your body as a whole.

DAN

Dan is a 34-year-old music composer who works long hours. He is self-employed and is super successful in his own right. Dan exercises five to seven times a week and does boxing, Pilates and high-intensity interval classes.

He came in to see me complaining of recurrent left-sided mid-back pain that radiated round into his left ribcage and also left chest area. He mentioned it was worse after he had been working for long hours and leaning across his equipment. I looked at his back and saw that there didn't seem to be too much structurally wrong, other than the fact that he had some muscle weakness in his shoulder and his breathing was quite shallow. Part of his spine didn't seem to be moving as well as the rest, so I worked with him to increase the movement and implement some exercises to encourage abdominal breathing and rib movements. I also encouraged him to try to set a timer on his phone to get up and move while working.

When Dan came back for his second appointment, he'd had no pain after his treatment for a few days, but it had gradually crept back. He then mentioned in passing, 'I had a bad weekend with food and drinking and I notice my back always hurts more when my IBS flares up too.'

This instantly made me think, 'Hang on a minute, this is no coincidence!' I then went on to ask him how often this happens and he said, 'Every single time I eat junk food and drink alcohol or my IBS has a flare-up, my back is bad. Every single time.'

I explained to Dan that it appears there could be a connection between his mid-back and rib pain, and his stomach problems and diet. I sent him to a nutritionist and she went through a plan with him.

I saw Dan about two weeks later after he had changed his diet. The nutritionist had asked him to cut out gluten from his diet and that was it. He came into clinic beaming and said, 'I've had no pain. Literally four days after cutting out gluten my back and rib pain went. If it creeps back, I then know I'm working for too long and I do some of the exercises you showed me.'

Dan does have gluten on the odd occasion and does experience the odd flare-up of his back. However, he now knows the cause and it means he can manage it better.

Could Your Eating and Drinking Habits Be Contributing to Your Back Pain?

Of course, there are times when things don't go according to plan, and there are a few habits I see in my clinics that can cause back pain . . .

Alcohol

Alcohol possesses both pain-relieving and anti-inflammatory properties, which may initially provide a sense of relief for people experiencing back discomfort. However, excessive or chronic alcohol intake can contribute to detrimental effects on overall health, potentially making pain worse. Alcohol can impair the quality of sleep, hindering the body's healing processes and potentially intensifying back pain over time.

In clinic I've had many patients over the years who have mentioned that after they've 'had a few alcoholic drinks' they notice that their pain levels are higher. Some theories postulate that the more alcohol you drink, the more it might exacerbate the pain you're feeling in your body. The reasons for this include:

- Dehydration: It is estimated that 70–80 per cent of your joint cartilage is made up of water.[43] Being dehydrated after alcohol may increase the pain felt in joints.
- Increase in inflammation: Some say that alcohol is broken down into toxic metabolites and this may increase inflammation throughout our bodies.

- Fatigue: Alcohol can make you feel quite sleepy and consequently this tiredness can make you feel generally lethargic and more achy than normal.

Try to drink responsibly and, when drinking alcohol, it's important to keep hydrated and try to ensure you get a good night's sleep. Current guidance from the NHS in the UK is for men and women not to drink more than 14 units of alcohol per week. To help you gauge how many units you're drinking:

- a single shot of alcohol = 1 unit
- a small glass of wine = 1.5 units
- one bottle of beer = 1.7 units
- one large glass of wine = 3 units

TIPS TO REDUCE YOUR ALCOHOL UNIT CONSUMPTION

- Track your intake: Keep a record of your alcohol consumption to be aware of how much you're drinking. This can help you identify patterns and make informed decisions about cutting down.
- Set limits: Establish specific limits for yourself, such as a number of drinks per day or week. Stick to these limits to ensure you don't exceed the recommended guidelines.
- Alternate with non-alcoholic drinks: When out socialising or at home, alternate alcoholic drinks with non-alcoholic ones like water, soda or mocktails. This can help slow down your alcohol consumption.

- Choose lower-alcohol-by-volume (ABV) options: Opt for beverages with lower alcohol content, such as light beers or wines with lower ABV. This can significantly reduce the number of units per drink.
- Be mindful of cocktails: Mixed drinks and cocktails can contain multiple types of alcohol and mixers, leading to higher unit counts. Be aware of the ingredients and their quantities in cocktails.

Caffeine

While caffeine intake is generally regarded as safe and may even offer some pain-relieving properties, excessive caffeine consumption may also have negative effects. High doses of caffeine can lead to increased stress levels, disrupted sleep patterns and heightened sensitivity to pain, potentially aggravating back discomfort. Moderate caffeine consumption could be considered as between one and three cups a day. You can try switching to decaf hot drinks and caffeine-free drinks as alternatives to help manage your pain levels.

Excessive salt intake

There is no strong evidence to suggest that salt intake is directly linked to back or muscle pain. However, excessive salt intake can contribute to several health problems that may indirectly lead to it. For example, a high-sodium diet can increase blood pressure, which can contribute to conditions like cardiovascular disease and kidney disease. These conditions can cause symptoms like back or muscle pain.

Additionally, excessive salt intake can lead to dehydration, which, as we'll come on to below, can cause muscle cramps and make it more difficult for your body to recover from exercise or other physical activity. This can also contribute to back or muscle pain.

It's important to maintain a balanced diet that includes a moderate amount of sodium, along with other important nutrients, to support overall health and reduce the risk of health problems that can contribute to pain.

What about sugar?

Again, there is no persuasive evidence to suggest that sugar intake is directly linked to back or muscle pain. However, a large amount of sugar can predispose you to several health problems, just like in the case of a high-salt diet.

For example, a high-sugar diet can lead to weight gain, which can put extra strain on the back and joints, leading to back or muscle pain. Additionally, a diet high in sugar can contribute to inflammation, which can also cause pain and discomfort throughout the body. Blood sugar levels can also impact pain. Diets high in processed sugar, in the form of things like cakes and sweets, will have an impact on our blood sugar levels, causing crashes and spikes. This plays havoc with our hormonal balance, which can worsen inflammation within our body and lead to an increase in back pain. Furthermore, consuming too much sugar can also lead to conditions like diabetes, which can cause nerve damage and contribute to conditions like neuropathic pain (when your nerves are damaged or not working properly – see page 39).

Below are my top three tips for avoiding high-sugar foods:

1. Read food labels: Check the nutrition labels on packaged foods. Look for terms like 'sucrose',

'high-fructose corn syrup' and other sugar-related terms. Choose products with lower sugar content.

2. Choose whole foods: Opt for whole, unprocessed foods like fruits, vegetables, lean proteins and wholegrains. These foods are generally lower in added sugars compared to processed and packaged items.

3. Cook at home: When you prepare meals at home, you have more control over the ingredients. This allows you to reduce added sugars in your meals.

OSTEO TOP TIP

When it comes to your eating habits and pain levels, it's important to pay attention to how your body responds to different foods. Grab a journal and a pen and write down what you've eaten over the last few days – as well as what you're about to eat. Go through and mark which foods you feel may be inflammatory and replace them with an alternative. For example, try replacing white pasta with wholewheat, have fresh fruit for breakfast or include plenty of different types of vegetables with your lunch or dinner. If you track your food over three days, you should be able to see if there's a change in your pain and therefore whether specific foods may be exacerbating your pain.

Hydration

A few studies have been conducted into the impact of dehydration on pain, and have shown that a lack of hydration can increase the pain sensitivity and pain stimuli within the brain.[44,45] There are also theories that suggest staying hydrated helps to keep the synovial fluid between our joints well lubricated, but this is an area that needs further research. Water is also considered to provide a great transport network through our lymphatic system, delivering healthy nutrients to our muscles and joints for healing in the case of an injury.

Severe dehydration typically presents as muscle cramps, extreme thirst and dizziness. However, just because you don't have the above symptoms doesn't mean you aren't dehydrated. Naturally, the more water you lose – for example, if you sweat a lot when walking or exercising, or simply live in a hot climate – the more likely it is that you will be dehydrated. Signs that you may need to add water to your diet include:

- Urine colour: Your urine should be light yellow or almost clear. The darker the yellow, the more water you may need to drink.
- Urine frequency: How often are you visiting the toilet? If you only go a few times a day, then it means your bladder isn't full enough to send the signal to urinate to your brain.
- Physical symptoms: Dry skin, mouth and lips may also be a sign of dehydration.

If any of these signs resonate with you, here are some easy ways to introduce more water into your life:

- Keep a glass of water on your bedside table or by your bed, so that when you wake up in the morning you immediately drink a glass of water.
- Try to drink a glass of water before lunch and dinner.
- Keep a glass of water by you at work to sip on.

- If you don't like the taste of water, you can add a squeeze of lemon or orange to it for some flavour.
- They say that people's brains make them feel hunger when actually it's more likely that they are thirsty. So before grabbing that mid-afternoon snack, try drinking a glass of water instead.

We should be aiming for eight glasses of water or 2–3 litres of water a day. Depending on how much you sweat you may require more than this.

Implementing Step 3: Eat Well

Now, this isn't a diet book – it's about pain in your body and giving you the tools to help yourself at home. However, I know that making changes to your diet can be tough and I see so many people in my clinics struggling to implement better lifestyle choices into their, often busy, day. I hear the same excuses week in, week out – and I get it. I want to empower you so you feel able to take control of your back pain, and I have therefore included my top tips below for overcoming these limitations:

The excuse: 'I don't have time'

This is a big one. It's one I use *all* the time. The truth is, though, I do have time. Of course I do! It really is just about what we prioritise. I'm guessing health is important to you, because you bought this book and you're actually reading or listening to it.

We know that ready meals are quick to prepare and consequently they are the easiest option for many of us who are time-poor. However, sometimes it's just about making better choices. We live in a world of convenience and things being portioned or premade for us. A perfect example of this is bags of salad, diced chicken breast, pre-cooked rice bags and pre-chopped onions or veg in the supermarkets. These can be a real saviour when you don't feel you have time in the day for food prep.

The most important thing, though, is to start small – implementing any of the small changes in the weekly plan below, even if you pick just one, can start to make the difference of feeding your muscles and joints with the best food.

The excuse: 'Healthy food costs a lot of money'

You know what . . . it doesn't *have* to be expensive. The branded items are always more expensive than supermarket own brands, but the taste is the same. Buying in bulk and freezing food is also a more cost-effective way to buy healthy, unprocessed food and not spend an absolute fortune at the same time.

The excuse: 'I like eating out a lot'

So do I! I love eating out – oh, the joy of having someone who chops stuff for me and puts it together in an effortless way is God's gift to my stomach. There is nothing wrong with eating at fast food or specialised dessert places. These foods in moderation are fine. However, sometimes we have to make some changes in order to feed our body with the correct nutrients for it to live its best life. Now, I know that some of you reading this are going to be saying, 'But I *have* to eat out for meetings or birthdays . . .' I get that, but there are definitely ways in which you can eat out but also make wise choices. Research restaurants online and check the menus for healthier, balanced options. Tell your friends or colleagues that you'll book the lunch or dinner venue so you're in control. Also there is a difference between eating out every day and eating out occasionally.

The excuse: 'Karen has no pain and she eats junk food all the time'

You are not Karen, and what Karen does is not relevant for you and your body. I get that it's easy to compare ourselves to our friends and to people on social media. However, we don't really know whether Karen is eating fast food ten times a day or whether she wakes up and runs 10km every single morning. In a nutshell, do not compare yourself to anyone else.

Try to remember that you are different and everyone's aches and pains and needs are going to be different. You don't know Karen's genetics, her underlying issues or what she does outside of her junk food lifestyle.

Next time you're on social media and fall into the trap of comparing yourself to someone else, concentrate on your breathing for 30 seconds. This will help to distract your mind, bring you into the present moment and get out of your thoughts. Unfollow or mute any accounts that you feel might be triggering your tendency to compare, and seek professional support if you find yourself regularly struggling with these thoughts on food and comparison (see Useful Resources, page 275).

The excuse: 'Healthy food tastes bad'

I often ask my patients to give me examples of the kind of foods they think are healthy and taste bad or boring. More often than not they say, 'low-fat butter', 'plain rice cakes' and 'calorie-counted/low-fat ready meals'. However, eating a balanced diet isn't about focusing on these bland 'low-calorie' or 'low-fat' foods, which are usually more processed than the original versions of the same products. When it comes to reducing back pain, it's about introducing more anti-inflammatory foods into your diet and getting a good balance of carbs, protein, fat, vitamins and minerals – and there is so much variety to choose from. A balanced diet has everything your body needs to stay strong and pain free, and you'll soon see that healthy food doesn't have to be bland.

Once you've overcome these barriers, below is a detailed weekly plan to help you see how you can gradually make changes to your diet.

Weekly plan

Week 1: Establishing the foundations

- Get planning: Buy a weekly planner for the fridge and plan your food for the week, so you know what you're eating when, and stick to it.
- Add one anti-inflammatory food, such as fatty fish, berries, leafy green vegetables, nuts or turmeric, to your diet each day. Try topping your cereal with some

berries, serving scrambled eggs with some wilted spinach or adding some turmeric into a stir-fry.

- Look back at page 159 and ensure each meal is balanced and contains the right quantities of carbs, protein, fat, fruit and veg.

Weeks 2–3: Mix things up

- Look at adding spices like cinnamon to your breakfast or turmeric to your lunch, and gradually increasing your fruit and veg intake to the recommended five a day.
- Take a little outing to the supermarket and look for the most colourful fruit and vegetables and try them.
- Replace sugary drinks with green tea or turmeric tea.

Weeks 4–6: Take it up a notch

- Buy and take supplements to augment your diet. I recommend curcumin, collagen and omega-3 (see page 163). Try intermittent fasting (see page 162) and see if it helps with your pain.
- Bulk-buy rice, chicken, tofu or similar healthy options, then spend some time portioning it up and putting it into separate bags in the fridge or freezer so you can grab it easily when you need to.

Weeks 7–8: Fine-tuning

- Block out time each week to meal prep food. Meal prep doesn't have to be complicated; it can be a simple salad or a bigger meal like beef chilli or chicken curry that you batch cook and then freeze.

- Try implementing one of the practical steps on page 170 each week to support your gut microbiome.
- Track your intake of alcohol, caffeine and sugar so you can identify patterns and cut down if necessary.

We know that pain is complex, but being able to identify foods that might be contributing to inflammation or gut dysbiosis can go some way to helping you heal your back. When looking at your diet, as with many things, it's about balance. We can't forget, though, that food brings lots of us joy and love! The areas I have covered in this chapter are a way of bringing new ingredients into your diet and recognising that a balanced, anti-inflammatory diet is a great way to fuel your well-being and your muscles – and reduce pain. Don't forget to track your progress weekly using the box above.

Rest and rejuvenation are also incredibly important when it comes to back pain and, in the next step, we'll be exploring how sleep impacts your back pain, with quick and easy tips to help you achieve a more restful night's sleep.

PROGRESS TRACKER

Remember to fill this in weekly, rating the following statements based on your experiences using a scale of 1–5, where:

1 = strongly disagree

2 = disagree

3 = neutral

4 = agree

5 = strongly agree

- Pain intensity: My overall level of pain has decreased.
- Daily activities: Pain has impacted my ability to conduct my usual daily activities.
- Mobility and flexibility: I have noticed improvements in my mobility and flexibility.
- Exercise consistency: I have been consistent with my exercises and physical activity.
- Core strength: I feel stronger in my core muscles, supporting my back.
- Stress levels: I feel more relaxed and less stressed.
- Mindset and attitude: I have noticed positive changes in my mindset and attitude towards managing my back pain.
- Nutrition habits: I have been able to maintain healthier eating habits focused on reducing inflammation.
- Overall well-being: I feel more confident in my ability to manage and alleviate my back pain.

CHAPTER 6

Step 4: Sleep Better

I HOPE BY now you've started to notice a real difference in your pain levels and have incorporated various tools and strategies into your week from the previous chapters. In this last step, we're going to look at sleep. This is a big one for many of my clients and it's something that we should all try to be a bit better at, regardless of our pain levels.

We all know that, when we've had a rubbish night's sleep – the kind of sleep that you keep waking up from and probably results in you getting fewer than six hours – our brain power and physical power are massively reduced and we function at a lower capacity.[1] In fact, research by Nuffield Health found that sleep disruption increases time off work by 171 per cent![2] When we are tired, lack concentration and have a low mood, this can also impact the way in which our body processes physical pain.

Lack of sleep and pain have one of those annoying relationships, where you don't always know what came first; lack of sleep can cause an increase in the pain you feel, and then the pain you feel increases the chance of you having a poor night's sleep. What is clear, though, is that addressing sleep issues can have a huge impact on how much pain you feel.

In this final step, we'll look at some simple ways in which you can catch a few more Zs and reduce your back pain. As you have done for the other steps, try to introduce a new sleep strategy each week and see if you begin to notice some changes in your sleep – and pain – over at least eight weeks. For those of you who suffer with pain every day and have done for a while, this might seem like a tough task, but it could be a key component to your recovery – so please stick with me. There is a weekly plan on page 220 to help you gradually incorporate the steps, and don't forget to monitor your progress with the tracker on page 221. Remember, a 'perfect' night's sleep may not be a straight eight hours, but it's something that works for *you* and makes you feel rested.

How Pain Impacts Sleep

Pain, specifically chronic pain, can have a big impact on both the quality and duration of sleep. One of the most common occurrences when it comes to pain and sleep is that sleep can be extremely 'broken' and those in pain can find themselves waking up repeatedly throughout the night. A person may find themselves awake for extended periods or experiencing frequent awakenings during the night, leading to a significant reduction in the quality and duration of their sleep. Not only is this frustrating when you're tired, but it will also have a direct impact on how quickly your back pain heals and, over time, can result in chronic sleep deprivation (a long time without sleep), which is associated with a range of negative outcomes, including an increased risk of depression and anxiety.

There are different stages in our sleep cycle and we need an equal balance of them all to wake up feeling rested and to help us to mentally and physically process the demands we place on our body during the day. These stages are referred to as light sleep, slow-wave sleep and rapid eye movement sleep. I don't know about you, but I can't go very long without sleep. I have always envied people who can function at work after having a few bad nights' sleep and still have energy. *I am not one of those people.* I need at least six hours' sleep to be able to hold a conversation and know what direction to walk in. I also know that I am not the happiest person to be around when I'm tired and that I can feel quite low. This is very common and, according to one study, around 75 per cent of people who are diagnosed as depressed also suffer from insomnia.[3] Things like anxiety and stress will have an impact on your sleep as well. There have been studies to show that conditions like sleep apnoea (when you stop breathing while sleeping) are also more prevalent in those with chronic pain.[4] In fact, come to think of it, if I am ever stressed and in pain (even if that's period pain), sleep is the first thing that suffers!

In addition, when you are in pain, your brain is active and aroused, which then keeps you awake. If this rings true for you, there are a few things you can do to calm your brain down, distract you from focusing on the pain and help you get some much-needed shut-eye. The exercises below are designed to be done most nights before bed. However, they're also good to do during the day if you want to. You could take 30 seconds at work and do them at your desk to have a mindful moment.

- Deep breathing: Put your hand on your abdomen and concentrate on breathing deeply so your tummy rises up and down slowly. This helps to relax your muscles and calm your nervous system. Focus on slow, rhythmic breaths to promote relaxation.

- Mindfulness meditation: Bringing yourself into the present can help to calm your nervous system down. You can do this by doing a body scan (see page 130) or even just saying the same positive sentence in your head over and over again for a few minutes (see page 144). Focus on your breath or sensations in your body, and let go of tension and anxiety.
- A relaxing bath: This can calm your mind and help you switch off before bed. A warm shower before bed can also help relax muscles.
- Light a candle: Lavender is a popular scent in modern sleep aids, like pillow sprays and temple rubs. However, it has been used for many years to help relaxation, so lighting a lavender candle before bed can be an effective way to relax the mind.
- Turn off your phone or avoid screens an hour before bed.
- Limit alcohol and tobacco use.[5]
- Pillow support: If you have lower back pain, place a pillow under your knees if you're lying on your back, or between your knees if you're on your side. This can help maintain the natural curvature of your spine and reduce pressure on your lower back.
- Do the pre-sleep mobility routine below.

PRE-SLEEP MOBILITY ROUTINE

1. Bring your knees to your chest and hold for ten seconds.
2. Sit on the edge of the bed and gently rotate as far as is comfortable to the left side and then the right.

---

3. Sit on the edge of the bed, make yourself into a small ball and then bend outwards and stretch.

4. Lie on the floor close to a wall and put your legs up against the wall. Your body will make an 'L' shape. Your hips can be against the wall or slightly away. Place your arms in any comfortable position. This pose has been shown to help with relaxation.

5. Lie on your side with your knees bent and your head on a cushion. Place your arms out straight in front of you. With the top arm, draw a circle around your body slowly and bring it back to sit on top of the other arm. Repeat this on both sides 5–10 times.

All of these things will set you up for a better night's sleep and help your body and your brain relax. If you have trouble getting back to sleep if you've woken up in pain overnight, the tips below might help:

- Gentle movement: Slowly change your sleeping position. Roll onto your side or back and make adjustments to find a position that provides relief. Avoid sudden or jerky movements.

- Stretching in bed: Perform gentle stretches while lying in bed. Bring your knees to your chest or gently arch your back to relieve tension. Avoid overstretching or straining your muscles.

- Heat or cold therapy: Apply a heating pad or cold pack to the affected area. Use caution to avoid burns or frostbite, and limit the application to 15–20 minutes.

- Over-the-counter pain relief: If you're comfortable with it and it's appropriate for your situation, consider taking an over-the-counter pain reliever as per the recommended dosage.

- Stay calm: Try to stay calm and avoid stressing about your back pain. As we saw in Chapter 4, stress can exacerbate the discomfort and isn't conducive to getting a good night's sleep. Remind yourself that you are taking steps to address the issue. You can also use the tips on page 127 to do some deep breathing to help calm you down.
- Avoid electronic devices: Resist the urge to check your phone or other electronic devices if you wake in the night. The blue light emitted by screens can interfere with your circadian rhythm and make it harder to fall back to sleep.
- Listen to relaxing sounds: Play calming music or use white noise to create a soothing environment. This can help distract your mind from the pain and promote relaxation.

Give these ideas a go and see what works for you – it's all about giving yourself and your back the best chance of getting the healing time you so desperately need!

How Sleep Impacts Pain

There is emerging evidence to show that sleep actually impacts the pain we feel more than the way in which pain impacts sleep. Poor sleep quality can have a significant impact on your body's ability to process pain. When you don't get enough restorative sleep, your body's pain threshold can decrease, making you more sensitive to pain. Additionally, lack of sleep can amplify the perception of pain, making it feel more intense. Studies have shown that a broken or short sleep time can mean that you have a heightened pain reaction and sensitivity to pain.[6] One study also found that poor sleep made lots of things worse, including pain, mood, range of motion and more.[7] It found that a poor night's sleep led to more pain at the start of the day than later in the day.

Our pain and sleep pathways cross over and melatonin, a hormone that regulates our circadian rhythm, has also been shown to have an impact on the *perception* of our pain.[8] Sleep deprivation or consistently not getting enough sleep may lead to a reduction in overall melatonin production. This can impact the ability to maintain a consistent sleep–wake cycle and may contribute to difficulties falling or staying asleep. In addition, melatonin influences the quality of sleep, so insufficient melatonin may result in lighter or broken sleep, reducing the healing benefits of rest. Sleep loss has also been shown to lead to an increase in inflammation within our bodies, which, as we've seen, may predispose us to feeling more pain.[9] Sleep is essential for the body's overall health and recovery processes. When you don't get enough sleep, your body's ability to heal and manage pain can be compromised.

People who are in chronic pain will feel super tired during the day because of their pain, and this will naturally mean that it's a struggle to follow a healthy exercise and movement routine, or choose a balanced diet, which can take time to prepare. And, as we're seeing with the four-step plan, these are all key ways you can help yourself out of the pain cycle by creating better habits and introducing small but impactful lifestyle changes.

Chronic pain also has a negative impact on mental health. Even though lack of sleep impacts pain directly, it also plays a role in mood and how we feel about ourselves. This low mood and negative mindset can also contribute to how we may experience pain and make it feel worse.

I know all this seems very doom and gloom – and it's so hard when you're in pain and it's affecting your sleep – but research has shown that good-quality sleep improves pain, and there are so many ways in which we can help to calm down the pain and increase the sleep.[10] Let's start with the position in which you sleep.

The 'Ideal' Sleeping Position

Many clients come to me saying that their sleeping position is causing their back pain – I hear it all the time. However, there is no concrete evidence to show this. In fact, there is more evidence to show that poor sleep categorically makes everything worse, so the most important thing is just to try to get some sleep, in whatever position you can.[11]

Having said that, lots of people struggle to find the most comfortable position to sleep in when they are in pain, so below are some tips that may help you avoid sleep positions that aggravate your pain:

- Pain on one side of your back: You might experience pain at night if you sleep on the same side as your pain. If this happens, try to avoid sleeping on this side.
- Lower back pain: There's some evidence to show that sleeping on your front can add pressure to your lower back.[12] As an alternative, you can try sleeping on your side with a pillow between your legs or on your back with a pillow under your knees.

- Nerve pain: If you have pain in your back and it also refers pain or pins and needles down your arms or legs, try to sleep on your back with a pillow underneath your legs or on your side with your knees slightly bent.

The research on sleeping positions just isn't conclusive enough to offer an 'ideal' sleeping position that suits every individual person, but in my own experience just concentrating on trying to get the best sleep you can, whatever the position, is the most important thing.

WHAT ABOUT PILLOWS AND MATTRESSES?

I get asked all the time what the best pillows and mattresses are. The reason for this is that people tend to blame the products they're sleeping on for their back pain.

In all honesty, when it comes to mattresses there is no one size fits all. Just as not all medications work in the same way for everyone, there is no one mattress that suits everyone. I often recommend that my patients go on an outing and try different mattresses in the shop. If this isn't an option for you, there are many online mattress companies now that allow you to try a mattress for a certain number of days, and you can send it back if it doesn't suit you.

Pillow choice is also very subjective. I have some patients who come in and say they don't sleep with any pillow and that their partner thinks that is 'bad for them'. The truth is, if your neck is fine and you're sleeping soundly, then it doesn't matter if you have no pillow.

MIKE

Mike came in to see me with left shoulder pain after injuring it playing golf. He described his pain as 'weird' as it felt like it was 'inside the joint', but he also had pain down the side of his arm, to about midway. This shoulder pain had started to aggravate an old back injury and so he was suffering with both when trying to sleep at night.

Mike showed me the sleep app on his phone and it revealed he had averaged about three to four hours' sleep a night over the past six weeks since the pain began.

When taking Mike's case history, I learned that he had a great exercise routine of walking to and from work, going to the gym to strength train three to four times a week and then also managing to do Pilates and yoga. He ate a well-balanced diet and was not overweight.

Mike told me that his main issue was that 'he couldn't sleep on his shoulder and couldn't sleep on the other side due to habit and his lower back pain'. He was told by another healthcare professional to 'never sleep on his front as it's very bad for your neck and lower back'. Mike was exhausted, frustrated and confused. He had also recently started taking the antidepressant sertraline as he had started to feel very low.

I treated Mike with shockwave therapy and some specific strengthening exercises to help support his shoulder and lower back. However, my main bit of advice to him was to sleep on his front. You can imagine his face – he was both shocked and happy. I explained to Mike that the most important thing was that he got 'the sleep'. Yes, he may experience a bit of neck pain or lower back pain when he woke up, but it was only because his body wasn't used to sleeping like that. It wouldn't cause any long-term damage or discomfort.

Mike came back two weeks later having followed my advice and once again showed me his sleep app. This time he had averaged seven to nine hours a night! And he reported a big improvement in his pain and his mood.

The Vicious Cycle of Sleep, Pain and Mental Health

As we explored in Part 1, pain is incredibly multifaceted and so it is important to consider the psychological factors that can impact your sleep, as well as the physical. Those who have chronic pain may feel like they are stuck in a cycle of pain, not being able to sleep and then feeling really anxious or depressed about it.[13] An example of how this might play out is you have pain and go to bed feeling anxious about your pain. The anxiety means you then can't sleep properly, have a disturbed night and wake up feeling more pain and more depressed.

When you have persistent back pain, this cycle can repeat for many nights. It can become overwhelming and you can end up catastrophising about it, as we explored in Chapter 4. You might find yourself thinking the worst and believing you will never get better. In fact, one study showed that people with osteoarthritis who catastrophised about their pain were more likely to experience pain than others.[14] Also it is no surprise that those in constant pain are more predisposed to going into a state of depression and can also get to a point where they are thinking about their back pain constantly. This can lead to poor sleep choices.[15] If this resonates with you, the exercise below can help you to break free from the cycle of catastrophising thoughts so you can get a good night's sleep.

Identifying negative thought patterns

Psychiatrist Aaron T. Beck created a model that is now widely used in cognitive behavioural therapy (CBT) treatments for negative thought patterns.[16] He created ten 'automatic thoughts' that often arise from various sources, including personal experiences, upbringing, cultural influences and cognitive biases. Take a look at the list below and I am almost certain that you will associate at least one of these with your back pain.

COMMON NEGATIVE THOUGHTS AND THEIR POTENTIAL SOURCES

1. Catastrophising: 'I need surgery on my back and will never walk again.'
   Description: Expecting the worst possible outcome.
   Source: Fear of failure, past traumas, anxiety.
2. Black-and-white thinking (all-or-nothing thinking): 'If this treatment doesn't work, then it means nothing will work for my back.'
   Description: Seeing things in extremes without recognising middle ground.
   Source: Perfectionism, rigid thinking, fear of ambiguity.
3. Overgeneralisation: 'I just felt a twinge in my back. Now I won't be able to move tomorrow and will be in agony no doubt.'

Description: Making broad, sweeping conclusions based on a single event.

Source: Traumatic experiences, low self-esteem.

4. Personalisation: 'I have back pain because I overworked myself in the gym; it's my fault and I deserve this.'

Description: Taking responsibility for events that are beyond one's control.

Source: Guilt, shame, low self-worth.

5. Filtering (selective abstraction): 'I know that I can tie my shoelaces now because my back is better, but I still can't play football and that's rubbish.'

Description: Focusing only on the negative aspects of a situation and ignoring the positive.

Source: Pessimism, past negative experiences.

6. Mind reading: 'The doctor thinks I'm lying about my back pain and that I don't know what I'm talking about.'

Description: Assuming you know what others are thinking and that it's negative.

Source: Insecurity, social anxiety.

7. 'Should' statements: 'I should be better by now and I should be training as I was in the gym.'

Description: Having rigid rules about how oneself and others should behave.

Source: External pressure, perfectionism.

8. Discounting the positive: 'I can get out of bed without pain now, but I still feel it in the base of my spine.'

Description: Dismissing positive experiences as irrelevant or unimportant.

Source: Low self-esteem, pessimism.

9. Emotional reasoning: 'I feel like this pain isn't getting any better.'
   Description: Believing that because you feel a certain way, it must be true.
   Source: Emotional distress, anxiety.
10. Labelling: 'My dad told me I'd get back pain like him and that means I'll now need surgery like he did.'
    Description: Assigning global, negative labels to oneself or others based on specific behaviours.
    Source: Low self-esteem, past criticism.

If you recognise some of these automatic thoughts, try recording them, their triggers and how you feel about them in a thought journal. Bringing awareness to your negative thought patterns and evaluating them in this way can help you feel more in control and gain insight into the areas you need to address. Simply writing down your automatic thoughts around your back pain can help reduce your anxiety and calm you down, which in turn will improve your sleep. It's also worth checking back to pages 140–142 for some tips on how to change your pain narrative and reframe your mindset.

Fear around bedtime

For those who experience difficulties with sleep, these can escalate into a full-blown fear or anxiety surrounding bedtime. There is a considerable body of evidence exploring the link between sleep disturbances and anxiety, with research highlighting the impact of both factors on mental health and pain.[17] As you can imagine, this is like a nightmare cycle for people who struggle with sleep and have back pain.

For some people, the fear or anxiety associated with bedtime can develop as a result of negative associations with sleep. If a person has experienced a traumatic event or excruciating pain in the past, they may associate bedtime with stress and anxiety, leading to a vicious cycle of sleep disturbances and anxiety. This can start a negative reinforcement cycle, where the individual becomes more and more anxious about going to bed, leading to even more sleep disturbance and further reinforcement of the anxiety. It is a bit like when someone has a fear of spiders. They will walk into a room and look for spiders in all the corners of the room because they are so scared, and therefore they are more likely to see them than someone who isn't aware of them. This is purely because the person who isn't scared doesn't look for them! When someone has had a bad experience with back pain at bedtime they can become hyperaware of the smallest niggles in their back that others with no back pain issues would ignore. This niggle can increase the anxiety around going to sleep and make restful sleep harder to achieve.

The impact of anxiety and fear around bedtime can be significant, with people experiencing a range of negative outcomes. These can include reduced quality of life, decreased productivity and increased risk of accidents or injuries. Some people often find themselves having to call in sick for work because exhaustion or lack of sleep has led to recurrent infections due to a lowered immune system. I have found that addressing sleep disturbances and anxiety together is the most effective approach, with interventions aimed at improving sleep quality also having a positive impact on anxiety symptoms. So it's all connected! If you can overcome this fear, you can then start to cement healthier sleeping habits.

OSTEO TOP TIP

Write a letter to your sleep. Yes, that's right. I want you to grab a piece of paper right now and write a letter to sleep and how you feel about it. This is going to enable you to go into your subconscious mind a bit more and recognise what might be causing your fear around sleep.

Your sleep letter might look something like this:

Dear Sleep,

I know we have had a temperamental time with each other. Sometimes I have no idea why you make me wake up and don't allow me to get back to sleep. I know that when I was little I used to get woken up by my parents arguing, but I am 35 years old now. I am over it . . . I think?

Maybe I'm not over it and maybe my subconscious has associated sleep with the trauma of my parents' divorce and how scared I was every bedtime. Either way, I know that we can have a better relationship and I want to work together to ensure that we can improve my health.

Love you lots,

Anisha

Some of the most effective treatments for anxiety-related sleep disturbances include CBT and relaxation techniques, such as meditation and deep breathing. These approaches focus on developing healthy coping mechanisms to manage anxiety and stress. Addressing these issues can have a positive impact on sleep quality, anxiety symptoms and therefore pain, improving overall mental health and well-being.

The strategies outlined in Chapter 4 will also support you in breaking free of this cycle and getting a better night's sleep. However, it is essential for those of you struggling with sleep disturbances and anxiety to also seek support from a healthcare professional like a doctor or sleep expert to develop an effective treatment plan tailored to your unique needs. This can also help reduce the likelihood of pain.

HEENA

Heena, a dedicated student with ambitious goals, came to see me feeling extremely frustrated with her back pain. She explained how 'the pain is making me feel so depressed. No one can tell me what is going on and I'm not sleeping and I have exams to pass.' She found herself caught in a cycle of back pain, disrupted sleep and declining mental well-being.

Heena's back pain led to her waking up in the middle of the night and struggling to get back to sleep again. This gradually became worse and her sleep became more broken and more uncomfortable.

Despite prescribed medication and rest, Heena's pain persisted, made worse by the ongoing battle with very limited sleep. Frustration grew as conventional remedies like painkillers and stretching made no difference. When she saw me she was really upset and I suggested CBT. Through a series of sessions, she learned to identify and reframe the negative thoughts and behaviours that were impacting her sleep and mood.

I also got Heena to do some mindful movement (see page 210) for five minutes before bed. These were slow and controlled, relaxing movements for her whole back. A combination of reframing her thoughts and mindful movement gradually reduced her pain and subsequently led to better sleep. This broke the cycle and also led to a much happier Heena, who wasn't in pain or sleep deprived.

How to Get a Good Night's Sleep When You're in Pain

As we've explored, poor sleep quality can lead to an increase in pain sensitivity and worsen symptoms, whereas good sleep quality can decrease pain sensitivity and help people cope better with their chronic pain. It's therefore so important to make sleep a priority. There is no magic wand here, but research has shown that better-quality sleep often starts with good sleep hygiene.[18] There are several things you can put in place to increase your chances of achieving a restful night's sleep, and therefore regulate your mood, reduce stress, increase your mental health and reduce your pain levels. Below are some simple strategies to consider when it comes to getting a good night's sleep when you are in pain.

Stick to a sleep schedule

Go to bed and wake up at the same time every day, even on weekends. This helps regulate your body's clock and can help you fall asleep and stay asleep more easily. Winning!

> **OSTEO TOP TIP**
>
> Use an alarm clock that recreates the sunrise. You can now get lamps that slowly lighten your bedroom in the morning. They can even recreate the sunset to help you fall asleep.

Create a sleep-conducive environment

Your bedroom should be cool, dark and quiet. Consider getting blackout curtains, an eye mask or earplugs to block out noise and light that may disrupt your sleep.

> **DON'T TAKE YOUR PHONE TO BED**
>
> Using your phone before bed can impact your sleep and, as we've seen, poor sleep can subsequently affect how your body processes pain. Here are some good reasons to leave your phone outside your bedroom and use an alarm clock instead:
>
> - Blue light exposure: Smartphones emit blue light, which can suppress the production of melatonin, a hormone that regulates the sleep–wake cycle. When you use your phone before bedtime, especially in a dark room, this blue light can trick your brain into thinking it's daytime, making it harder to fall asleep.
> - Delayed sleep onset: Engaging with your phone before bed can be stimulating and mentally engaging, which can delay the onset of sleep. This

delay can lead to a shorter overall sleep duration and less restorative sleep.
- Increased stress and anxiety: Scrolling through social media or reading news updates on your phone before bed can expose you to stressful or anxiety-inducing content.

Put away your phone or screens an hour before you go to bed.

Develop a bedtime routine

Doing calming activities before bed, such as taking a warm bath, reading a book or practising relaxation techniques, like yoga or deep breathing, can help signal to your body that it's time to wind down and prepare for sleep. Try to do this at the same time every night if you can.

WHAT YOUR BEDTIME ROUTINE COULD LOOK LIKE

Here's a step-by-step example of a bedtime routine, including approximate times:

- 9.30pm: Start winding down. Begin your bedtime routine about an hour before you plan to sleep. This gives your body and mind time to relax and prepare for sleep.
- 9.30–10pm: Dim the lights. Lower the overall lighting in your home or bedroom. Bright lights can inhibit the production of melatonin, the hormone that helps regulate sleep.

- 10pm: Disconnect from screens. Turn off electronic devices such as smartphones, tablets and computers.
- 10–10.30pm: Engage in calming activities. Choose activities that help you relax and unwind. This could include reading a book, listening to soft music, practising gentle stretching or yoga, or taking a warm bath or shower.
- 10.30pm: Prepare your sleep environment. Ensure your bedroom is conducive to sleep. Make sure the room is cool, quiet and comfortable. Consider using blackout curtains, earplugs or a white noise machine if necessary.
- 10.30–11pm: Practise relaxation techniques. Incorporate relaxation techniques into your routine. This might involve deep breathing exercises, progressive muscle relaxation or meditation. These techniques can help calm your mind and prepare your body for sleep.
- 11pm: Settle into bed. Get into bed at a consistent time each night. Create a relaxing pre-sleep ritual, such as applying lotion, sipping herbal tea or writing in a gratitude journal. Avoid stimulating activities or discussions at this time.
- 11pm–7am: Sleep time. Aim for a consistent sleep schedule by allowing yourself at least 7–8 hours of sleep each night. Stick to the same wake-up time, even on weekends, to regulate your body's internal clock.

Watch what you eat and drink

Those who struggle with broken or deprived sleep for a long period of time can become dependent on caffeine during the day to help them cope with the exhaustion. However, it's important to avoid large meals, caffeine and alcohol before bed. These can interfere with sleep quality and make it harder to fall and stay asleep. Try to eat at least one hour before you lie down. If you can't do this, you may experience bloating and feel uncomfortable, which can make it harder to fall asleep.

SLEEP-SUPPORTING SUPPLEMENTS

Magnesium has a natural calming effect on your body and mind, making it easier to relax and fall asleep. It also works with a chemical in your brain called GABA, which helps reduce feelings of anxiety and promotes relaxation. Magnesium is important for making melatonin, a hormone that tells your body it's time to sleep. It can also help relax your muscles, relieving any tension or cramps that might keep you awake. Lastly, magnesium can help reduce stress and anxiety, making it easier to unwind and get a good night's sleep. If you're having trouble sleeping, trying magnesium supplements or talking to a healthcare professional might be worth considering.

Melatonin is a hormone produced in our pineal gland and it's important for regulating our circadian rhythm. Melatonin supplements are used as a short-term aid for those experiencing jet lag and can also be helpful for those suffering from sleep problems, such as insomnia.

Many of my clients use these aids to help them relax and consequently have a better night's rest.

Get regular exercise

Physical activity can help promote better sleep, but avoid exercising vigorously too close to bedtime as this can be stimulating and make it harder to fall asleep. Even though it's tempting to do exercise before bed when you are stuck for time, try to replace any quick workouts with slow, controlled mobility exercises like Pilates or yoga. These are still good for you, but are less likely to get your blood pumping.

> **MINDFUL MOVEMENT**
>
> Mindful movement is when you are *present* while you are doing your exercises. You are thinking about where you are placing your hands and which parts of your body you are stretching or strengthening. You are also breathing while you move. The combination of mindfulness and movement helps reduce cognitive distraction, in that it brings you into the present, increasing both physical and mental relaxation. This should help you to have an easier sleep onset.

Don't take work into the bedroom

I know it's unavoidable for some people, but try to work in a different room in your home if you can. Alternatively, go to a coffee shop or other public working space such as a leisure centre if available. If you have to work in your bedroom and can fit a desk in, work from there and not from your bed. Make sure to turn off your computer at the end of the working day and put it away if possible, so you're not tempted to check emails after hours. The bed should only be used for two things: sleep and getting jiggy with it.

Manage stress

As we explored in Chapter 4, stress and anxiety can interfere with sleep, so finding ways to manage stress throughout the day can help promote better sleep at night. Try relaxation techniques, such as meditation or mindfulness, or talk to a therapist or counsellor if needed. Meditate for a few minutes before bed to calm your mind and be present. Try not to always rely on your phone for guided meditations. You can also find a mantra that you repeat ten times to help calm your mind.

WHAT IF YOU STILL CAN'T SLEEP?

If you are struggling to get to sleep, get up. Don't lie there with your eyes open thinking about how flies don't migrate to hotter countries in the winter. More importantly, try to avoid the temptation to scroll in the middle of the night or open specific apps. Instead, move to a different space or try another activity like cleaning or ironing, then, when you feel sleepy, go back to bed and try to sleep again.

Consider sleep aids or medication as a last resort

If you're still having trouble sleeping despite making these changes, talk to your doctor about sleep aids in the form of medication. However, these should be used as a last resort and only under the guidance of a healthcare professional.

ELIZABETH

Elizabeth, 70, came in to see me with chronic back pain that she'd had for the last ten years. Her back was impacting her daily activities and she had decided that it was unlikely to get better; she came to see me as a 'last attempt' at trying to help it.

On chatting with Elizabeth, I discovered that ten years ago she had got an electronic tablet. This was something that she enjoyed playing games on for hours and hours at night. She said she would often get lost in the game and then realise it was 2am and struggle to 'switch off'.

I didn't want to take away Elizabeth's joy of playing games, so we compromised with her playing in her living room on the sofa only. We agreed that she wasn't to take screens into her bedroom as she had a house phone in case of an emergency.

Not only did Elizabeth later report less pain in her back, she also said that she was getting a better night's sleep. By changing the location of where she played her games, it helped her sleep better and that in turn helped her back. She initially refused to believe that such a simple swap would help her, but I always like proving people wrong. For the right reasons obviously!

Anisha's bedtime back pain routine

Below is the bedtime back pain routine I give to my patients in clinic. Many find this routine makes a real difference to their back pain overnight and therefore their overall sleep.

Of course, one of the challenges I see my patients facing is time. I completely understand that you won't want to do a 30-minute routine for your back pain every night before bed, especially when you're in pain and tired, so I've included three variations for you. Use these as you wish, though obviously the longer you can do, the more likely you'll be able to ease yourself into sleep. These routines incorporate a combination of movement, mindset and sleep. Feel free to adjust the timing of each activity based on your personal preferences and needs.

Routine 1 (5 minutes)

1. Mindful breathing (2 minutes): Sit comfortably on the edge of your bed, close your eyes and focus on your breath. Inhale deeply through your nose, hold for a moment and exhale slowly through your mouth. Repeat for a couple of minutes.
2. Gentle stretch (2 minutes): Perform a simple seated forward fold. Sit on the edge of your bed, extend your legs and reach forward. Feel a gentle stretch in your back and hamstrings. Then put your feet back down and twist round to the left and right.
3. Mindful chanting or affirmations (1 minute): Softly chant a calming phrase or repeat a positive affirmation. Focus on the soothing sound and let it bring tranquillity.

Routine 2 (10 minutes)

1. Prepare your space (1 minute): Set the mood by dimming the lights and ensuring a comfortable room temperature.

2. Mindful breathing (3 minutes): Begin with a mindful breathing session in a comfortable seated position, focusing on deep, intentional breaths.
3. Gentle stretches (4 minutes): Incorporate the seated forward fold, cat-camel stretch (see page 104) and child's pose (see page 57) to release tension in the back. These movements should be slow and controlled.
4. Mindful chanting or affirmations (2 minutes): Engage in mindful chanting or affirmations to shift your focus and promote relaxation.

Routine 3 (30 minutes)

1. Prepare your space (2 minutes): Take time to create a calming atmosphere with dim lights and a comfortable room temperature.
2. Mindful breathing (5 minutes): Begin with a mindful breathing session in a comfortable seated position.
3. Gentle stretches (10 minutes): Explore the seated forward fold, cat-camel stretch, child's pose and legs-up-the-wall pose (see page 192) for a more extended release.
4. Mindful chanting or affirmations (5 minutes): Dedicate a few more minutes to mindful chanting or affirmations to deepen the sense of tranquillity.
5. Journalling (5 minutes): Take a few minutes to write down what's in your head in a notebook.
6. Final relaxation (Savasana) (3 minutes): Lie down, close your eyes and focus on your breath during a final relaxation period.

Understanding Pain on Waking

Before we close this chapter, I want to address something that is extremely common: pain when waking up in the morning. I hear 'I woke up with it' almost every single day in my clinic. This isn't just about back pain, of course – it's about many conditions like neck pain, headaches, plantar fasciitis (inflammation of the base of your foot), Achilles tendinopathy, carpal tunnel syndrome, repetitive strain injury, osteoarthritis and more.

Waking up with back pain, or any other kind of joint pain, is very rarely a serious issue. However, I do understand how upsetting it can be when you wake up with pain in the mornings. Both acute back pain (sudden-onset, sharp pain) and chronic back pain (constant, dull ache) seem to like taking us poor sleepy humans by surprise in the mornings. In fact, some of my clients report being pain-free during the day and only having pain when they wake up in the morning.[19]

Morning back pain is often frustrating as it is another one of those 'unexplained' things. It is hard to comprehend that doing nothing and being at rest has caused pain, and then most people associate this pain as being damage or bad for them and 'can't understand why it has happened'. Often it might spiral into the catastrophising behaviour we explored earlier: 'Goodness, I can't even rest or sleep and wake up and feel better. My back is doomed. I probably have arthritis everywhere.'

I can see why and how people think like this. It's unfair right? It's unfair that all you did was sleep and the next-door neighbour plays football, rugby and goes to the gym and has zero injuries or problems (as far as you know anyway).

So, what causes morning pain? Chronic (long-term)

morning back pain is difficult to pinpoint as, like with chronic back pain generally, it probably has a number of causes. However, there are some explanations as to why morning back pain seems to be a 'thing'.

Cause number 1: Sleeping awkwardly

Sleeping awkwardly isn't about poor posture at night. They are two different things. Poor posture is thought of as being a slumped-over, lazy posture and is considered to be 'your fault', whereas an awkward posture is basically falling asleep with your arms above your head like a princess, or with your ankle up by your ear, or something ridiculous that isn't your fault as you're unconscious. If you sleep in one of these awkward positions, you might be there for a long period of time and this can cause pain on waking.

Our bodies like to move and any forced stagnant posture is going to contribute to more pain.

Cause number 2: Inflammation in your body and back

There are more severe back conditions that can cause back pain, like spondyloarthritis and AS, which are classified as autoimmune inflammatory diseases. The umbrella term is typically 'inflammatory back pain'. These conditions are often very severe and consistent in the mornings, but they are also more likely to wake you up in the middle of the night. They are also related to other symptoms such as inflammation in other body parts including joints, tendons or your digestive system, a family history of autoimmune diseases and/or an infection prior to the morning back pain developing.

However, there is also a general increase in slow and mild inflammation as we age. Often you will notice as you get older, or people around you get older, that they complain of their joints aching or they groan when they get out of bed because they feel stiff. They often attribute this to disc degenerative changes or arthritis, but it's not often the case. It is more likely to be widespread inflammation over the entire body.

The cause of widespread inflammation might be metabolic syndrome, which is an umbrella term used for a condition in people who don't do much exercise, might be overweight and have long-term stress.[20] It's also known as 'inflammageing' as there is evidence to show that, regardless of how fit, healthy and lean you are, you're still going to have some slow, gradual inflammation throughout your body as you age.[21]

I've outlined some ways in which you can combat this below – you'll see that we've already touched on some of these in earlier chapters.

1. Eat a healthy, balanced diet, which involves not limiting yourself to particular foods and making sure you have a combination of protein, carbohydrates and healthy fats in your diet (see Chapter 5).
2. Invest in your sleep – we now know the power.
3. Build your strength with exercise and movement (see Chapter 3).
4. Decrease your stress levels by participating in more mindfulness techniques and seeing your friends often (see Chapter 4).
5. Take anti-inflammatory medication – we know this might help widespread inflammation in your body, but not everyone likes to take medication. The one thing I will say is that it does prove to be a useful diagnostic tool. If

your symptoms and morning pain reduce as a result of taking the medication, then it's a good indication that inflammation is probably the cause of your discomfort.

Cause number 3: Fibromyalgia

This is a condition with several symptoms, including fatigue, widespread joint pain and muscle aches, mental confusion and exercise intolerance. Many of these symptoms are a cocktail for pain and consequently the lack of sleep, tiredness and lack of exercise are going to contribute to feeling back pain in the morning. Diagnosing fibromyalgia can be difficult as other conditions have similar symptoms, such as fatigue, low mood and aches and pains. If you suspect that fibromyalgia may be the cause of your morning pain, it's important to see your doctor so they can rule out other underlying conditions and give you an official diagnosis.

Cause number 4: Vitamin D deficiency

We saw how important vitamin D is in the last chapter, but vitamin D deficiency is common in about one in six people in the UK.[22] If you are deficient, you may experience widespread pain and discomfort. It can cause bone aches and pain in the back, which may be felt more in the morning.[23]

Vitamin D deficiency is also known as osteomalacia, which is essentially softening of the bones due to not having enough vitamin D. If you feel you may be deficient in vitamin D, see page 165 for tips on how to increase your intake.

If you wake up and find your back is sore and stiff, try my morning mobility routine below.

ANISHA'S MORNING MOBILITY ROUTINE

1. While lying on your back in bed, bend your knees slowly and gently rock them from side to side within your pain threshold. Try to get further very gradually so that you're getting some rotation through your spine. It may take a few minutes to get comfortable to push that stretch.
2. One by one, slowly bring each knee to your chest. Put your hands around your knee and pull it towards your chest.
3. Pull your tummy in, keep breathing normally, lift up your pelvis and slowly turn onto your side. From this position you can gently shuffle to the edge of the bed and use your arms to sit up.
4. Once you're sitting on the side of the bed with your legs off the side, gently rotate left and right as far as you can, slowly for about 30 seconds. You should then be able to stand up. It might still be a bit painful and sore, but remind yourself that your body is strong.

(Please note: In the unlikely event that you have any loss of sensation in your legs or numbness around your pelvis and genitals, please call the emergency services.)

Implementing Step 4: Sleep Better

Below are my quick wins when it comes to increasing your sleep (and therefore reducing your pain), followed by a weekly plan if you need some more guidance.

- Light exposure: Get exposure to natural light during the day, especially in the morning, to regulate your circadian rhythm.
- Limit naps: If you nap, keep it short (20–30 minutes) and avoid napping late in the day.
- Create a sleep-friendly schedule: Align your schedule with your natural circadian rhythm. Go to bed and wake up at the same time every day.

Weekly plan

Week 1: Establishing the foundations

- Bedroom set-up: Ensure your bedroom is cool, dark and quiet. Consider using blackout curtains and earplugs. Check your pillow and mattress are right for you.
- Sleep schedule: Set a consistent bedtime and wake-up time, even on weekends.
- Evening routine: Wind down 30 minutes before bed with calming activities such as reading a book or taking a warm bath.

Weeks 2–3: Creating healthy sleep habits

- Limit screen time: Avoid screens (phones, tablets, computers) at least one hour before bedtime and don't take your phone to bed.
- Regular exercise: Engage in regular physical activity. Try my bedtime back pain routine on page 212.
- Be mindful of your diet: Avoid heavy meals, caffeine and alcohol close to bedtime. Stay hydrated, but limit liquid intake close to bedtime to minimise broken sleep.

Weeks 4–6: Reducing stress

- Deep breathing: Focus on slow, rhythmic breaths to relax your muscles and calm your nervous system.
- Try relaxation techniques: See if meditation or mindfulness help to calm your mind and reduce racing thoughts.
- Meditate: Meditating for a few minutes before bed can help to bring you into the present and aid with getting a good night's sleep.

Weeks 7–8: Consolidation

- Write a letter to your sleep: Try the activity on page 203 to address any fears you may be holding around sleep.
- Keep a thought journal: Make a note of any automatic thoughts you have around sleep and pain, and their triggers, and see page 199 for tips on how to feel more in control of your negative thought patterns.
- Supplements: Try sleep-supporting supplements such as magnesium or melatonin (see page 209).

I hope that the small changes you've started to make have made a difference to your sleep and you've noticed a positive shift in your pain levels too. Remember, building new habits takes time, but it really pays off in the long term – and consistency is key. Keep tracking your progress using the box above and be motivated by all you have learned about the crucial role sleep plays in the overall health of your spine and managing and preventing back pain. Taking these simple, practical steps can change your pain and your life.

Next, as we transition to Part 3, we'll explore the treatment options that might be right for you, as well as how to overcome any obstacles you may have faced along the way, so you can make these steps a sustainable part of your lifestyle.

PROGRESS TRACKER

Remember to fill this in weekly, rating the following statements based on your experiences using a scale of 1–5, where:

1 = strongly disagree

2 = disagree

3 = neutral

4 = agree

5 = strongly agree

- Pain intensity: My overall level of pain has decreased.
- Daily activities: Pain has impacted my ability to conduct my usual daily activities.
- Mobility and flexibility: I have noticed improvements in my mobility and flexibility.
- Exercise consistency: I have been consistent with my exercises and physical activity.
- Core strength: I feel stronger in my core muscles, supporting my back.
- Stress levels: I feel more relaxed and less stressed.
- Mindset and attitude: I have noticed positive changes in my mindset and attitude towards managing my back pain.
- Nutrition habits: I have been able to maintain healthier eating habits focused on reducing inflammation.
- Quality of sleep: I have experienced improvements in the quality of my sleep.
- Overall well-being: I feel more confident in my ability to manage and alleviate my back pain.

PART 3

What Next?

I am hoping you've got to this point in the book and you are feeling empowered and able to take on the *world!* OK, maybe not the world, but maybe just your body and the pain you've been experiencing.

By implementing small but gradual changes from the four steps in Part 2, I hope you have begun to see powerful results and now understand just how incredible your body is.

In this last part of the book, we'll look at treatment options for when you have back pain, so you can decide what is best for you, as well as how you can troubleshoot and ensure all your hard work isn't undone.

CHAPTER 7

Treatment Options

LOTS OF CLIENTS come to see me having been diagnosed with a severe back condition such as disc degeneration or a disc prolapse. I know this can be a daunting experience, often accompanied by significant pain and discomfort. However, it's important to recognise that such a diagnosis doesn't necessarily equate to an immediate need for surgery. Manual therapies (like osteopathy), targeted exercises, pain management strategies and lifestyle modifications can often play a crucial role in improving one's quality of life and reducing discomfort. In fact, you will already have gone a long way in healing your back pain by dedicating yourself to the four steps outlined in Part 2.

Before we discuss the different treatment options available on both the NHS and privately, it's important for you to be aware of something known as the 'outcome of interest'.

Identifying Your Outcome of Interest

The 'outcome of interest' refers to the specific health outcome that medical care aims to achieve for each patient. In other words, it is the measurable result of medical care that is most important to the patient and healthcare provider. The outcome of interest can vary depending on the medical condition being treated and the goals of the individual patient.

For example, if you have lower back pain, your outcome of interest may be to be able to get out of bed without pain in the morning or bend down to pick up your child. This is the most important thing when it comes to treatment options as we're focusing on your desired outcome.

Now, I know a lot of you will be thinking, 'My desired outcome is pretty obvious – I want to have no pain and never have to think about my back ever, ever again, even when I'm 85!' I get it, but what is more realistic is your 'why'. Let's break it down with an exercise:

OSTEO TOP TIP

Grab a notebook or digital device and write down three things that will make you realise your back is strong. For example, 'Picking up my kids and not thinking about it', 'Putting on my socks easily' or 'Playing tennis again'.

These are your outcomes of interest – your measurables – and it is our job as clinicians to work *with* you to make these happen, or to be realistic about how close you can get to them.

With back pain, go towards what you want and not away from what you don't want.

Ultimately, your outcome of interest is super important because it helps to guide treatment decisions, assess the effectiveness of interventions and evaluate the overall quality of care that you might be receiving. By focusing on your outcome of interest, healthcare providers can tailor their approach to meet your specific needs and optimise your personal health outcomes. This approach ensures that medical care is focused not just on treating the possible disease, but also on improving your quality of life and achieving the best possible health outcomes.

REMEMBER: EVERYONE IS DIFFERENT

People's bodies are different. What works for one person may not work for another. Factors like genetics, lifestyle and overall health play a role in how quickly a person's body responds to an injury and how it heals. Think of it like cars: different makes and models need different kinds of maintenance during the car's lifespan.

The type of back pain also matters. Some injuries, like a simple muscle strain, might heal faster than a more complicated problem involving discs or nerves. Again, if we compare our bodies to cars, it's a bit like comparing a minor scratch on your car to a deeper mechanical issue.

Try not to compare your recovery with someone else's – keep in mind your outcome of interest and what it means for you, personally, to heal your back.

Now that you know your 'why', you can go to your healthcare provider confident in the knowledge of what you want to achieve that is specific to you. They can then help get you there. The next step is understanding the different treatment options available and which might be right for you. Remember, though, it's crucial that you get a proper diagnosis from a medical professional before embarking on any treatment journey.

Non-Invasive Treatment Options

Often my clients don't want to have invasive treatment, they don't like the thought of needles or want to do things as naturally as possible without taking medication. While sometimes medication and surgery are necessary, in many cases non-surgical treatments and therapies can effectively manage and alleviate the symptoms associated with back pain. Surgical intervention is typically considered when conservative measures prove ineffective or in cases of severe neurological impairment, which is when the nerves are affected in a way that cannot be solved by manual therapy. So, while the diagnosis may be concerning, there is often a range of non-invasive treatment options available to explore – many of which, such as osteopathy, acupuncture, physiotherapy, shockwave therapy and exercise classes, are available on the NHS – before resorting to surgical procedures.

Massage

Some people hate massages and some love them. I lean more towards the latter, and many of my clients ask me whether they should have a massage between osteopathy sessions. My answer is, if they want one, then of course!

There isn't enough evidence to show that anything physical happens when a muscle is massaged. However, massage therapy clearly has some benefits, otherwise we wouldn't all love it. Maybe this has something to do with touch, but massage therapy can also help promote relaxation and reduce stress levels, which, as we explored in Chapter 4, can contribute to the development and exacerbation of back pain. By reducing stress and promoting relaxation, massage therapy can help alleviate the psychological and emotional aspects of back pain, which can, in turn, lead to decreased physical symptoms.

Overall, the evidence suggests that massage therapy is a safe and effective intervention for reducing back pain.[1] Regardless of whether something is going on biologically or not, pain is being reduced and people are feeling good. So having a massage isn't going to do you any harm, in my personal opinion.

WHAT ABOUT SCAR TISSUE MASSAGE?

Scar tissue occurs when we are cut or have had a trauma that created internal damage – for example, back surgery on a herniated disc or a C-section when having a baby (this can impact back pain as there is decreased support to the spine and increased strain on the back muscles as they temporarily compensate for the weakened abdominal muscles). Scar tissue is part of our body's healing process to bring the tissues back together and it is formed of collagen. There are many massage therapists who provide 'scar tissue' massage and there is evidence to show that this can really help the pliability, pigmentation and pain of scar tissue.[2]

Acupuncture and dry needling

Acupuncture involves inserting thin needles into specific points on the body to alleviate pain and promote healing.

While the exact mechanisms by which acupuncture works are not fully understood, there is mounting evidence to suggest that it can be a safe and effective treatment option for back pain. For example, a review of 29 randomised controlled trials found that acupuncture was significantly more effective than no treatment for chronic back pain.[3]

Acupuncture is a popular form of treatment on the NHS for musculoskeletal pain for this reason. However, many people are worried about needles and therefore don't feel happy undergoing this form of treatment. If this is you, let me share an interesting fact: an acupuncture needle is about a quarter of the width of an ordinary needle – about the thickness of a thread – so it's unlikely you will feel any pain.

One of the key benefits of acupuncture is its ability to stimulate the release of natural pain-relieving chemicals in the body, such as endorphins and serotonin. Acupuncture may also help to reduce inflammation and improve circulation, both of which, as we've seen, can contribute to back pain relief. Like anything that involves lying down and stopping for a bit, it will also help reduce cortisol levels and enable you to be more present and mindful, which, as we saw in Chapter 4, can also alleviate pain.

It's worth noting that there are several different types of acupuncture, each with its own unique approach. Traditional Chinese acupuncture, for example, is based on the concept of balancing the body's energy flow (or 'qi') through the use of needles inserted into specific points along energy pathways known as meridians. This form of acupuncture is based on traditional Chinese medicine principles and is often used to treat a wide range of health issues, including pain, stress, anxiety and digestive disorders.

In contrast, dry needling is a relatively new technique that was developed in the West and is primarily used to treat pain and musculoskeletal conditions. Dry needling involves inserting thin needles into trigger points or knots in muscles to release tension and relieve pain. The technique is based on the modern understanding of neurophysiology and musculoskeletal anatomy, rather than traditional Chinese medicine principles.

Another significant difference between acupuncture and dry needling is the way in which the needles are inserted. Acupuncture needles are typically inserted at specific depths and angles, and may be left in place for several minutes to promote energy flow. Dry needling, on the other hand, involves inserting the needles directly into trigger points or tight muscles, often with a quick in-and-out motion.

While the specific type of acupuncture used may vary, skilled acupuncturists will work with the patient to identify the underlying causes of their pain and develop a treatment plan that is tailored to their unique needs and goals, and this usually takes their whole lifestyle into consideration.

Whichever form of acupuncture you choose, finding a qualified practitioner who can provide personalised care is essential for achieving the best possible outcomes.

Transcutaneous electrical nerve stimulation (TENS)

A TENS machine is a device that sends electrical impulses through the skin to stimulate nerves and reduce pain. The exact mechanism of how TENS works to reduce back pain is not fully understood, but there are a few theories:

1. Gate control theory: According to this theory, the electrical impulses from the TENS machine block the pain signals from reaching the brain by stimulating

the nerves in the area where the pain is felt. This creates a kind of 'gate' that blocks the pain signals, reducing the perception of pain.

2. Endorphin release: TENS may also work by stimulating the release of endorphins, which are natural painkillers produced by the body. Endorphins can help reduce the perception of pain and promote a feeling of well-being.

3. Increased blood flow: TENS may also improve blood flow to the area, which can help reduce inflammation and promote healing.

Though more research is needed to fully understand its effectiveness in treating back pain, a systematic review and meta-analysis of 24 randomised controlled trials found that TENS was effective in reducing chronic lower back pain, with no significant adverse effects reported. The authors concluded that TENS could be a safe and effective treatment option.[4]

Shockwave therapy

Shockwave therapy is a non-invasive medical treatment that uses high-energy acoustic waves to stimulate healing in various conditions, such as musculoskeletal and soft tissue injuries, plantar fasciitis and tendinopathy. The evidence for shockwave therapy on pain is mixed and depends on the specific condition being treated and the amount of time a person may have been suffering with the condition they are presenting with.

For example, shockwave therapy has been shown to be beneficial for conditions such as tendinopathy, reducing pain and improving range of motion. However, the evidence in other conditions such as tennis elbow and Achilles tendinopathy is less clear. Some studies have shown significant pain reduction with shockwave therapy, while others have found no difference compared to placebo treatments. As with many other treatment methods, shockwave therapy requires more research to be carried out. However, when I have used shockwave therapy on my clients in clinic, I have noticed a big improvement in their recovery from back pain.

Manual therapy

Manual therapy is a type of hands-on treatment that is often used to relieve musculoskeletal pain and improve mobility. There are several different types of manual therapy, each with its own unique techniques and approaches.

Here are some of the most common types of manual therapy and their main differences:

1. Chiropractic manipulation: This involves using a high-velocity, low-amplitude force to manipulate the joints of the spine or other parts of the body. Chiropractors use this technique to help relieve pain, improve mobility and restore normal function. I guess chiropractors are famous for getting the best 'cracking' sounds from joints.

2. Osteopathic manipulation: This type of manual therapy is similar to chiropractic manipulation. Osteopathic manipulation typically involves gentler, more rhythmic movements that aim to improve circulation and restore balance to the body.

3. Physiotherapy: Physiotherapists or physical therapists use a variety of manual techniques to help improve mobility, reduce pain and restore function. This may

include joint mobilisation, soft tissue mobilisation and manual stretching. They often do exercises with the patient to help strengthen specific muscles.

4. Myofascial release: This technique involves applying sustained pressure to specific points in the body to release tension in the fascia. I would say that all types of manual therapists, including osteopaths, chiropractors and physiotherapists, use this type of treatment.

Each type of manual therapy has its own unique benefits and limitations, and the choice of which technique to use depends on your individual needs and condition. It's also worth mentioning that these therapies now overlap, and many physiotherapists use manipulation and many osteopaths and chiropractors offer exercise rehabilitation advice. This is why, when I am interviewed on the television or in publications, I am more inclined to talk about the similarities rather than the differences between these therapies – we are allied and work together.

THREE MYTHS ABOUT OSTEOPATHY

1. You're going to be in agony after treatment: Some people might experience soreness after a session, but this is often not classed as agony.
2. You will be told to stop doing activities that you love: It's highly unlikely your osteopath will tell you to completely stop moving. As we saw in Chapter 3, movement is good for you! It's more likely we will adapt your movement for a bit and then get you back to where you want to be as soon as possible.

> 3. You'll be given lots of exercises to do that take too long: It's our job to make exercises manageable within your lifestyle and routine. We will do our best to tailor exercises around your time constraints to ensure you are still improving.

Manual therapists explore and take medical case histories of their clients and approach these cases on an individual basis. They do this by including the following practices:

- Exercise therapy: Exercise therapy is a key component of physiotherapy for back pain. There is strong evidence that exercise therapy can improve pain, function and quality of life in people with chronic back pain.[5] The specific exercises prescribed will depend on the individual's condition, but may include stretching, strengthening and aerobic exercises.
- Mobilisation techniques: There is moderate evidence that techniques such as spinal mobilisation and manipulation can provide short-term relief of pain and improve function in people with chronic back pain, and clients do report an improvement in their symptoms.[6]
- Education and advice: Manual therapists can provide education and advice on back pain management, including postural awareness, ergonomic adjustments and activity modification. There is strong evidence that patient education can improve outcomes in people with back pain – and this is my main aim with this book![7]
- Other methods: Manual therapists may also use various methods, such as heat or cold therapy, electrical

stimulation or ultrasound, to help manage pain and improve function.

No one profession is better! We all have the same desire in mind, and that is to help our patients achieve their outcome of interest, whether that is jumping on a trampoline with their kids or jumping out of a plane. We share the same goal, and that is for everyone who walks through our doors to live their best life.

CHOOSING A MANUAL THERAPIST

Choosing who to see for your back pain can feel quite overwhelming. Fear not – the tips below should help you find the right therapist for you.

1. Think about your network of friends, family or colleagues. Have they been to see someone about their back pain? If so, it might be worth asking them for a recommendation. Make sure to ask a few people, though, as they will have differing opinions or you might find the same name comes up repeatedly.
2. Local groups on sites like Facebook often allow you to ask for recommendations in your area.
3. Always check reviews, both on search engines and the therapist's website itself. This will give you a good indication of the quality of treatment and results you will receive.
4. If you are still unsure who to see, you can also call the clinic you would like to visit and ask them, for example, whether their therapists can treat lower back pain or the difference between a

---

physiotherapist, osteopath and chiropractor. Listen for how friendly and informative they are. Most clinics have a team that should be able to answer these questions in a neutral tone.

5. Lastly, the distance to the practice can be relevant when you're experiencing a particularly sore flare-up. Commuting for treatment that's quite far away may cause more discomfort or stress, which may not do your back any favours!

Reiki and energy healing

Reiki is a form of energy healing that is based on the concept that the practitioner can channel healing energy into the recipient's body to promote balance, relaxation and overall well-being. Reiki is believed to work by clearing blockages in the body's energy field, which can lead to physical, emotional or spiritual imbalances.

Scientifically, the concept of an energy field or life force that can be manipulated for healing purposes is not well understood or supported by current scientific evidence. However, some studies have shown that reiki can reduce stress and anxiety, increase relaxation and feelings of well-being, and improve various physical and mental health outcomes, which, as we've seen, can all have an impact on pain levels.[8]

I often get asked by my clients about reiki and it is something that I have always found fascinating – my science osteo brain doesn't quite get it, but my 360-degree approach to well-being really does. Overall, while the scientific evidence for reiki and other forms of energy healing is limited, many of my clients report positive experiences and benefits from these therapies.

Hydrotherapy

Hydrotherapy is a therapeutic approach that involves the use of water for pain relief and other health benefits. Hydrotherapy can take many forms, such as soaking in a hot tub, taking a warm shower or bath, or using a cold compress.

One of the most common forms of hydrotherapy is the use of warm water, which can help to relax muscles, increase circulation and reduce pain and inflammation. Warm water can also promote relaxation and reduce stress, which can further contribute to pain relief and overall well-being.

While more research definitely needs to be carried out, studies have suggested that warm water immersion in hydrotherapy can cause blood vessels to dilate, leading to increased blood flow to the affected areas.[9] This increased blood flow can help to deliver oxygen and nutrients to the muscles, while also carrying away metabolic waste products that can contribute to muscle soreness and fatigue.

Cold-water therapy

Ice baths and cold showers are having a bit of a moment. Whether it's on TikTok or Instagram, cold-water immersion has become a health-related trend, but what do we know about it?

Ice baths involve immersing the body in very cold water, typically between 10 and 15°C, for a short period of time, usually 10–15 minutes. Ice baths are often used by athletes to help reduce inflammation and promote recovery after intense workouts or competitions.

A more accessible option for many people is having a cold shower. A blast of cold water at the end of your shower has also been shown to reduce inflammation and relieve localised pain.[10] Remember to take it slow – start with a 30-second blast and then work up to one or two minutes gradually.

There has been some evidence to support the following benefits of cold-water therapy when it comes to pain:[11]

- Release of endorphins: Cold-water exposure can trigger the release of endorphins, which are natural painkillers and mood boosters.
- Reduction in inflammation: Cold-water immersion has been shown to reduce inflammation in the body, which can help to speed up recovery from muscle soreness and injuries. This is due to the parasympathetic branch being activated, which calms you after a stressful event (see Chapter 4).
- Improved circulation: Once you get out of a cold shower or ice bath, the blood vessels in your skin dilate, which can improve circulation and promote healing.

At the time of writing, I have zero desire to immerse myself in an ice bath. However, people often describe ice baths like 'coffee on steroids' and many of my clients report feeling amazing afterwards and super awake and energised. It's a big adrenaline rush and some people love that, while others don't.

Like everything, there are risks associated with essentially shocking your body with cold water. People with certain medical conditions, such as Raynaud's disease or heart problems, should avoid cold-water exposure. Additionally, prolonged exposure to cold water can be dangerous and even lead to hypothermia, so please consult with a medical practitioner before giving it a go yourself.

Lower back braces

There are many types of back supports out there, but the most common one I see my patients using is lower back braces. So, what do lower back braces do?

- They increase the feeling of spinal support, which will encourage more confidence and therefore movement.
- They increase your intra-abdominal pressure (the pressure inside your belly, created when your abdominal muscles tighten during activities like breathing, lifting or coughing). This pressure provides stability to your spine, protects your internal organs and helps in various body movements.
- They may help with power and speed.
- They reduce the stress on the spine when doing certain movements.

It's also important to understand that back braces *don't*:

- prevent any injuries
- cause your core muscles to weaken
- prevent a reduction in range of movement
- provide support to your spine

However, in my opinion, you probably don't need a back brace. They can inhibit lymphatic drainage in the injured tissues and, from my experience, should only be used when absolutely necessary – such as after surgery or an extremely acute bout of back pain. As we explored in Chapter 1, your spine and lower back are super strong. It's best to get to the root of the problem and not become dependent on supports.

LESS PAIN = MORE PRODUCTIVITY

If you're in pain or sore, then it's safe to say that you're probably going to be distracted at work, and this can mean you're unable to focus fully on the task in front of you.

Though not a treatment option in itself, I want to highlight the importance of having an active workplace set-up that encourages movement while you're working. Some of the most common reasons people experience pain at work can be due to lack of movement and using unsupportive equipment. An office desk chair without lumbar support, or a desk that is too high or low, for example, can contribute to injury and existing conditions.

Sometimes the joints need to have some rest, and using things like a supportive keyboard and ergonomic mouse can help to reduce the amount of movement through the wrist and elbow joint. This not only helps to reduce any aches or pains, but also manages stress when it comes to wanting to keep working.

Psychological Treatment Options

In Chapter 4 we explored how our emotions can impact pain, and there are various ways in which psychological treatments might help with pain. Below I cover the kinds of therapies that are available and the techniques they use in order to help you manage your mindset and pain.

CBT

CBT is a form of psychotherapy that focuses on helping you identify and challenge negative thought patterns and beliefs about your pain and develop more positive coping strategies.

Some examples of CBT techniques that may be used include:

- Cognitive restructuring: This technique involves the therapist helping you to examine the evidence for and against your negative thoughts and beliefs, and develop more balanced, realistic alternatives (like the reframing exercise you did on page 141).
- Relaxation training: This technique involves relaxation techniques, such as progressive muscle relaxation or deep breathing exercises, to help reduce pain-related tension and anxiety.
- Behavioural activation: This technique involves encouraging you to engage in enjoyable activities, even if you are experiencing pain. This can help to improve mood and reduce the focus on pain.
- Graded exposure: This technique involves gradually exposing you to activities that you may be avoiding due to fear of pain or injury. The therapist helps you to develop a plan to gradually increase your activity level, with the goal of increasing function and reducing pain-related disability.

Acceptance and commitment therapy (ACT)

ACT is a form of therapy that aims to help people accept difficult thoughts and feelings while also working towards their values and goals. It can be used to help develop a more accepting attitude towards pain, while also taking steps towards improving overall quality of life. It is a flexible and adaptive approach to helping people cope with pain.

Some examples of ACT techniques that may be used include:

- Mindfulness: Mindfulness techniques, such as mindfulness meditation or body scans (see pages 126 and 130), can help people become more aware of their thoughts and emotions related to pain, and develop a more accepting attitude towards these experiences.
- Values clarification: ACT emphasises the importance of identifying and clarifying our values and acting towards those values even in the presence of pain. The therapist may help you identify meaningful activities and goals and develop a plan to pursue those goals despite pain.
- Cognitive diffusion: This technique involves helping people to separate themselves from their thoughts, and to view them as simply thoughts rather than absolute truths. This can help to reduce the impact of negative thoughts related to pain.
- Acceptance: ACT emphasises the importance of accepting difficult thoughts and feelings related to pain, rather than trying to avoid or suppress them. The therapist may help you to develop a more accepting attitude towards pain, while also taking steps towards improving your overall quality of life.

Mindfulness-based stress reduction (MBSR)

MBSR is a programme that teaches how to use mindfulness meditation and other mindfulness techniques to reduce stress and manage pain. It can be used to help people become more aware of their thoughts and feelings related to pain and develop a more mindful and accepting attitude towards their pain. This is more to teach people the different ways to practise mindfulness. We've already explored mindfulness meditation in Chapter 4, but some other MBSR techniques include:

- Yoga: MBSR incorporates gentle yoga postures and movements, which can help to improve flexibility, strength and balance. Yoga can also help to cultivate mindfulness, as you focus on the sensations of movement and breath.
- Mindful movement: This technique involves bringing mindfulness to everyday movements, such as walking or eating. The goal is to develop a greater awareness of the body and the present moment in everyday activities.
- Group support: MBSR is often taught in a group setting, with opportunities for people to share their experiences and receive support from others. This can help to foster a sense of community and connection, which, as we saw in Chapter 4, can be important for managing stress and chronic pain.

Hypnotherapy

Hypnosis has been used as a complementary therapy for managing pain for many years. It is believed to work by altering a person's perception of pain, which can reduce the intensity of the pain experience. The exact mechanisms of how hypnotherapy works are not yet fully understood, but it is thought to involve several processes. For example, hypnotherapy may activate the parasympathetic nervous system, which, as we saw in Chapter 4, is responsible for the body's relaxation response, and promote feelings of calm and relaxation. It may also help to reduce the activity of the sympathetic nervous system, which is responsible for the body's stress response.

Hypnotherapy may also work by changing a person's beliefs, attitudes and perceptions about their pain or condition. For example, it can help to reframe negative thoughts and emotions that contribute to pain and discomfort, and replace them with more positive and constructive ones.

There is evidence to support the use of hypnosis for pain relief, although the results can vary depending on the individual and the specific type of pain being treated. A meta-analysis of 18 studies involving over 900 patients with chronic pain found that hypnosis was associated with significant reductions in pain intensity, pain unpleasantness and anxiety compared to control conditions.[12] Additionally, brain imaging studies have shown that hypnosis can influence activity in the areas of the brain associated with pain processing, suggesting that it may work by modulating the brain's perception of pain.

Overall, while hypnosis may not work for everyone or for all types of pain, there is evidence to support its use as a complementary therapy for pain management.

Medications

Topical treatments

I often get asked my opinion on over-the-counter ointments for back pain. Many of them are heavily advertised on the television and online as being an effective way of reducing your pain.

There are various topical creams, gels and balms for back and muscle pain on the market, ranging from complementary therapies to non-steroidal anti-inflammatory drugs (NSAIDs). Let's look at a few of the most common ones now.

Arnica gel, despite its popularity, lacks substantial evidence supporting its ability to treat pain. Tiger balm tends to provide a soothing warmth (verging on a burning effect), but also contains ingredients such as camphor that can divert your attention from pain. It is this distraction that instils a sense of confidence to then engage in more movement. As we covered in Chapter 3, we know that movement can really help to reduce your back pain.

Back rubs, such as Deep Heat, claim to increase the blood supply to the area and therefore relax and soothe the muscles. However, the jury is still out on whether this actually happens. The rub might have warming properties, but it may not necessarily increase blood supply. It is thought that the warming effect may be a placebo and make people feel less pain.

Cooling sprays or gels are similar to Deep Heat in that they may not do anything physically to the muscles, but they can provide a sense of distraction and relief that may help with the confidence to move.

When it comes to cannabidiol (CBD) oils and balms,

there's not enough research on them as yet, but the research that has been done shows that they could be beneficial in reducing back pain.[13]

Diclofenac gels, such as Voltarol, are topical NSAIDs that specialise in addressing superficial inflammation and prove to be quite effective in treating specific injuries locally. There have been trials on the use of diclofenac as an ointment that show it can penetrate the skin by up to 1cm, which may help reduce the pain in a muscle.[14] However, most of these studies need further testing to ensure their results are valid. The advantage of these gels lies in their targeted application, avoiding the need to inundate the entire body with medication. Voltarol can be a valuable tool for joint pain and superficial inflammation, offering targeted relief. However, it's crucial to stress the importance of obtaining a proper diagnosis before embarking on any treatment journey. While Voltarol is great at managing inflammation, it's important to remember that, in cases of back pain, the presence of pain doesn't always correlate with inflammation.

This is where the steps outlined in Part 2 come into play, providing alternative strategies to effectively address any type of back pain. In my experience, if topical ointments are providing you with the ability to have some confidence in the strength of your back and consequently encouraging you to move more, then that can only be a good thing.

Painkillers

I mean, the name itself is pretty enticing, isn't it? No one likes pain, so the idea of killing it is great. Different types of painkillers work in different ways. For example, aspirin and ibuprofen work by blocking the production of chemicals called prostaglandins, which are involved in inflammation and pain. Other painkillers, like paracetamol (also known as acetaminophen), work by blocking pain signals that travel along nerves to the brain. When we feel pain, it is because the nerves in the affected area send a message to the brain telling us that something is wrong. These painkillers block these messages, so even though the problem is still there, we don't feel the pain as strongly or at all. Stronger painkillers, like opioids, work by binding to specific receptors in the brain and spinal cord to block pain signals.

Painkillers can be effective in reducing pain and inflammation associated with back pain, and they can improve your quality of life by allowing you to move more freely and participate in activities that you enjoy. However, the use of painkillers should always be discussed with a qualified healthcare professional, as there are potential risks and side effects associated with their use. Painkillers are good at helping with the fear that can sometimes be created by experiencing pain, but they also need to be used cautiously in the event of a serious injury. For example, it's not advisable to fall over while skiing, break your shoulder and take painkillers in order to mask the pain to keep skiing for the rest of the week, as it could potentially lead to more complications (this is a real story that a client told me!).

NSAIDs, such as ibuprofen or naproxen, are a common type of painkiller used to treat back pain. They work by reducing inflammation and pain, and can be effective for mild to moderate pain. However, long-term use of NSAIDs can increase the risk of gastrointestinal problems, such as ulcers and bleeding, and can also affect kidney function. It is important to use NSAIDs as directed and to avoid taking them for prolonged periods of time without medical supervision.

Paracetamol is generally considered safe when used as directed, but can cause liver damage when taken in high doses or in combination with alcohol.

Opioids come with a high risk of addiction and other serious side effects, and should only be used under medical supervision. Patients should be closely monitored for signs of dependence or overdose.

CBD

CBD has become a bit of a buzzword in recent years. It is often used as a natural remedy for pain relief, but it is not typically considered a traditional painkiller or analgesic like aspirin or ibuprofen. Rather, CBD is believed to work by naturally reducing inflammation in the body and it may also reduce anxiety levels, which can in turn alleviate pain.

CBD is known to interact with the body's endocannabinoid system, which is involved in regulating a wide range of bodily functions, including pain perception. By interacting with cannabinoid receptors in the body, CBD may help to reduce inflammation and pain.

It is important to note that much of the evidence on CBD is still preliminary, and more research is needed to confirm its potential benefits and to better understand any potential risks or side effects.[15] Additionally, the regulatory landscape around CBD can be complex, as it is still not fully legal in all jurisdictions and its legality can vary depending on the source and concentration of the CBD.

JAMES

James came to see me in clinic with ongoing left-sided back pain. He suffered with this after sustaining a football injury and then deciding to play football again. He didn't have much fear around his pain, so this meant that he rested for a while and then played sport again. However, you need to allow adequate time to recover and rest before going back to the sport you love. We discovered that James maybe went back to sport a bit too soon.

He asked me what my thoughts were on CBD oil and I told him that he was free to try it if he wished, and that some people report amazing benefits and some don't. (Which is the truth with most things – honestly, we are so individual.)

James decided to buy some CBD oil and take it every night before bed. He came back to see me eight weeks later and was absolutely 'buzzing' about CBD. He explained how he felt less stressed, was sleeping better and his occasional back pain was virtually gone.

Quite often, as we've seen in previous chapters, the fact that CBD helps many things like anxiety and sleep will also have an impact on pain levels, so it might be something you want to discuss with your healthcare professional.

Further Treatment Options

If the non-invasive treatments outlined above aren't right for you or haven't had the desired effect, your healthcare practitioner may recommend further exploratory interventions, which we'll look at now.

To scan or not to scan? That is the question

When they're in pain, have tried multiple avenues to try to get answers as to why they're experiencing it and have tried various treatment options, it is no surprise that one of the first things my patients say to me is, 'Do you think I should get a scan?'

Now, don't get me wrong, MRI scans are amazing! MRIs were developed to be able to see each and every structure within our bodies. They can be immensely beneficial in specific scenarios and provide much-needed reassurance to those experiencing pain or discomfort, helping to rule out severe underlying conditions and providing a clearer understanding of the issue. Additionally, MRI scans can be essential in managing expectations regarding recovery time, particularly when dealing with conditions that require patience, as prolonged discomfort can lead to impatience and low mood, which can, in turn, exacerbate pain. In cases of acute injuries, such as an ankle sprain, MRI scans offer a precise view of the extent of damage, aiding healthcare professionals in devising the most effective rehabilitation plan – this facilitates a quicker return to sport and normal activities.

However, while scans may offer some answers for some people, there is also evidence to show that they may not be as beneficial and useful as expected.[16] MRI scans are not infallible and can sometimes yield results that are not entirely accurate. False positives or false negatives can occur, leading to unnecessary concerns or missed issues.

The decision to have a scan for back pain depends on several factors, including your specific symptoms, clinical findings and the judgement of your healthcare professional. It's important to consider the evidence regarding their usefulness for back pain:

- Acute non-specific lower back pain: For those with acute non-specific lower back pain (pain that is not caused by a specific underlying condition – see page 48), routine imaging is generally not recommended. Multiple studies have shown that routine imaging in these cases does not improve outcomes or lead to better treatment decisions.[17] Most cases of acute lower back pain resolve on their own within a few weeks with conservative management and by following the steps outlined in Part 2.
- Red flags: Red flags are warning signs that may indicate a more serious underlying cause of back pain, such as infection, tumour, fracture or spinal cord compression. In the presence of red flags like unexplained weight loss, history of cancer, severe trauma or neurological symptoms, imaging is usually warranted to identify or rule out these serious conditions.
- Chronic lower back pain: In cases of chronic lower back pain (pain persisting for more than 12 weeks – see page 46), the decision to undergo imaging depends on the clinical judgement of the healthcare professional. Research suggests that imaging findings, such as degenerative changes or disc herniations, are often present in asymptomatic people as well.[18] Therefore, imaging alone may not provide a clear explanation for the pain or guide treatment decisions.

- Progressive or worsening symptoms: If the individual's symptoms are progressive, worsening or not responding to conservative management, imaging may be considered to assess for specific causes, such as spinal stenosis, disc herniation or spondylolisthesis (see page 253). In these cases, imaging can help identify structural abnormalities that may require targeted interventions.

It's worth noting that unnecessary imaging can lead to additional costs, incidental findings that may cause unnecessary anxiety and potentially unnecessary interventions or surgeries. Therefore, the decision to have a scan should be based on a careful evaluation of your clinical presentation and the potential benefits versus risks of the procedure.

Incidental findings refer to unexpected or unintended findings discovered during imaging tests that are unrelated to the reason for which the test was performed. These findings can include abnormalities, lesions or anatomical variations that were not the primary focus of the imaging study.

Several studies have examined the psychological impact of incidental findings.[19] Some research suggests that those who receive incidental findings experience heightened levels of anxiety, distress and concern about their health compared to those who do not receive such findings.[20] The uncertainty surrounding the significance and potential consequences of the finding can contribute to this heightened anxiety. Furthermore, incidental findings can lead to a cascade of further tests, consultations and interventions, which can also contribute to increased anxiety and stress. The need for additional investigations or medical interventions can add to the emotional burden and uncertainty experienced by people, which can exacerbate any pain. Collaborative decision-making and involving patients in the process can help alleviate this anxiety by empowering them to be active participants in their care.

ANTHONY

Anthony, a computer technician, came to see me in clinic with ongoing lower back pain. He had been to see another therapist previously and they advised him to have an MRI on his entire spine. This MRI showed that Anthony had slight disc degenerative changes in his lower back, but the thing that he was most concerned about was that the scan showed he had a disc prolapse in his mid-back.

He didn't have any mid-back pain at all, but his anxiety went through the roof, and it started to affect his sleep and stress levels. Consequently, his lower back pain seemed to get worse as well and he came in confused, upset and scared.

I spent some time with him to explain that many disc prolapses don't result in symptoms (see page 19) and that they happen more often than people realise. I reassured him that he was strong and didn't have anything to worry about with regards to his mid-back. By slowly getting him to work on his anxiety and helping to empower him, his sleep improved, his stress levels reduced and his back pain disappeared.

I now see Anthony once a year and he's working out regularly and running the marathon later this year.

Steroid injections

Steroid injections, also known as corticosteroid injections, involve the administration of an anti-inflammatory medication directly into the painful area of the spine. This form of treatment is commonly advised when more conservative measures, such as manual therapy and oral medications, have proven ineffective at addressing pain and inflammation associated with certain spinal conditions like spinal stenosis, disc herniation and facet joint arthritis. The purpose of these injections is to reduce inflammation and pain, and enhance the overall function and movement of the affected region.

Laser therapy

Laser therapy, also known as low-level laser therapy or cold laser therapy, involves the application of low-intensity light to the affected area of your back and spine. Laser therapy may increase cellular activity by increasing blood flow and promote healing processes within the surrounding tissues. While the exact mechanisms of how this works are still undergoing research, there is suggestion that laser therapy may enhance blood flow and reduce inflammation and pain. The research around laser therapy for back pain is evolving and the results are mixed.

Surgery

Surgery is considered a last resort in the management of back pain and is usually only recommended when conservative measures have proven ineffective and there is structural damage (for example, disc herniation) or pathology (for example, cancer) that requires intervention.

The most common back pain surgery includes a discectomy (removal of a herniated disc), laminectomy (removal of the lamina to relieve pressure on the spinal cord) and spinal fusion (joining two or more vertebrae together). These surgeries are aimed at addressing specific structural issues contributing to pain and discomfort.

Things that influence the decision for back surgery by professionals include the severity and duration of symptoms, the presence of neurological symptoms (like nerve referral down the leg) and the failure of more conservative treatments. Surgery, when deemed necessary by experts (orthopaedic and/or neurological surgeons), can offer relief and improve the quality of life for those struggling with persistent and debilitating back pain.

An example of how surgery may be warranted and beneficial is actually from my own personal experience. In 2016 I injured my left wrist, which felt catastrophic at the time. After conservative efforts failed, we discovered I had something called a positive ulna variance, which is when the ulna bone in my arm is longer than it should be. As it was a structural defect, it required intervention with surgery to shorten the bone (ulna osteotomy). This was scary, especially as my hands are my livelihood. The rehab process was long and I had to be patient, but one year after surgery I was back lifting weights in the gym, including doing pull-ups. I thought I wouldn't be able to treat patients again, but the surgery changed everything for me.

With this in mind, I want to reassure those of you who have been told they will require surgery on their back that consultants and doctors would only do this as a last resort and they have extensive knowledge of what will help reduce your pain and improve your quality of life. The outcomes of these surgeries can be life-changing and, although daunting, often have phenomenal results.

Treatment for Acute Injuries

For a long time, RICE – rest, ice, compression and elevation – was considered the first thing you should do for an acute injury, such as a fall or a sprained muscle. We would see physios or doctors running up to athletes with a bag of ice cubes for an injury. However, the latest research shows that, even though putting an ice pack on an injury can have analgesic effects (like a painkiller), it is often short term.[21]

There is now a more holistic and balanced approach. Created by physiotherapists Blaise Dubois and Jean-Francois Esculier in 2019, the PEACE and LOVE acronym has replaced RICE and is now considered to be the best way to treat an acute sprain or injury.[22] Here's what each letter stands for:

PEACE:

- Protection: Protect the injured area from further damage or stress. This might involve using a brace, crutches or other supportive devices.
- Elevation: Elevate the injured area above the heart to help reduce swelling and improve blood flow to the area.
- Avoid anti-inflammatories: Avoid the use of anti-inflammatory drugs or other methods that might interfere with the body's natural healing process.

- Compression: Use compression to help reduce swelling and support the injured area.
- Education: Seek out education and guidance from a healthcare professional or athletic trainer on how to best manage your injury and promote healing.

LOVE:

- Load: Gradually introduce loading and stress to the injured area to help promote healing and restore function. This might involve gentle exercises, stretching or other activities that gradually increase in intensity over time.
- Optimism: Maintain a positive outlook and focus on the progress you're making rather than getting discouraged by setbacks or delays in healing.
- Vascularisation: Encourage blood flow and circulation to the injured area through gentle movement, massage or other techniques that can help promote healing.
- Exercise: Engage in exercise and physical activity that supports your recovery and helps restore strength, flexibility and function to the injured area.

Overall, the PEACE and LOVE approach encourages protection and support for the injured area while also promoting healing, restoration and the long-term ability to function.

What about heat?

Without a doubt, heat is popular when we are in pain or have aches. The number of clients I see who tell me that they've been having a hot bath every day or using a hot water bottle to help ease their pain is far higher than those who use an ice pack or ice bath.

Heat therapy works by increasing blood flow and circulation to the affected area, which can help relax muscles and alleviate pain. Heat can also help reduce stiffness and improve flexibility, which can be particularly helpful for those with chronic back pain. There is some evidence to suggest that it can be beneficial for reducing pain and promoting healing.

A systematic review of 21 randomised controlled trials found that both superficial heat (such as hot packs or warm-water baths) and deep heat (such as ultrasound or diathermy) were effective for reducing pain and improving physical function in people with non-specific lower back pain. The review also noted that heat therapy was a safe and low-cost treatment option for back pain.[23]

I hope the information you have read in this chapter has helped you think about which treatment option might be right for your own back pain, and which might help you to achieve the outcome of interest you identified on page 227.

All of the steps in Part 2, as well as these treatment options, are great for when you're at the height of your pain. However, I know from speaking to my patients that, sometimes, it's hard to get started with self-care practices or to continue with them when pain flares up unexpectedly, so the next chapter is all about troubleshooting and showing you how making small changes and being consistent are key to healing your back.

CHAPTER 8

Troubleshooting

DEPENDING ON WHERE you are on your journey to healing
your back, you might now be at the point where you've
incorporated some of the strategies from each of the four
steps, your pain has considerably eased and you feel empowered
by your new knowledge. This is great – well done for
committing to making changes to your diet and sleep, as well
as implementing stress-reduction techniques and introducing
movement into your day. In my experience, clients who
continue to commit to these small lifestyle changes see the
most benefit with regards to their pain in the long term.

It may be that you've been taking the steps one at a time
and have made a start with introducing gradual movement
throughout your day, for example, but have yet to make
tweaks to your diet or try stress-reduction techniques such as
mindfulness or meditation. That's OK too – everyone is
unique, and for these changes to have a real impact on your
pain you need to feel that you're doing things in the way you
need to. You do you! In time, you'll realise that all these little
changes become a natural part of your life and you won't
have to consciously implement them.

I'm very aware, too, that some of you may have struggled
to implement any of the strategies outlined in Part 2. I see this

occasionally in my clients and so want to take some time now to explore any barriers to change you may be facing.

Overcoming Barriers to Change

It is essential to recognise whether any of the barriers below are hindering you from actioning the steps outlined in Part 2. Identifying your barriers to change can help you to develop strategies to overcome them and increase the likelihood of making positive changes in your life – and therefore reducing your pain.

Lack of motivation

Sometimes, people know what they need to do, but they lack the motivation to follow through with it. This could be due to various reasons, such as feeling overwhelmed, experiencing depression or anxiety, or simply not seeing the benefits of taking action.

The fix: Find a friend who already engages in the habits that you would like to integrate and ask to go with them to a Pilates class or the gym.

Start with small or even tiny steps to make the change. You don't have to go all in from the start. Maybe take a five-minute walk around the house or the block and then gradually build that up.

Fear of change

People may resist change, even if it is positive and beneficial, because it disrupts their current routine and comfort zone. They may worry about the unknown or fear losing control of their lives. The reason we all like our comfort zones is because we don't really like uncertainty and want to feel safe. Routine and pattern provide that security for us and is less stressful. When it comes to back pain, it can be quite scary. This can initiate fear avoidance, where you feel too scared to try something new or something that you know may aggravate your symptoms.

We are all creatures of habit and it's normal to feel unsettled by change. However, if you can take some steps to overcome this, it can make a big difference to your back pain.

The fix: Quite often, gradually starting to introduce the movements that you are fearful of can help strengthen your body and remind your brain of how strong it is. So going slightly out of your comfort zone is sometimes all it takes.

Grab a notebook or digital device and write down all the reasons you want to make this change and why you bought this book in the first place. Read it over and over again to remind yourself that the fear is normal, but will not serve you in helping to heal your back.

Negative self-talk

Sometimes, people engage in negative self-talk, where they doubt their abilities and criticise themselves for not being able to follow through. This can lead to feelings of shame, guilt and anxiety, which can further decrease motivation and self-esteem.

The fix: Your beliefs can be changed if you work to recognise where they have come from and use the tools in Chapter 4 to reframe your mindset. If you need further support, see the

Useful Resources on page 275 for some recommended charities or organisations that can help.

Lack of accountability

When people do not have someone holding them accountable, such as a coach, therapist or friend, it can be easy to fall back into old habits and resist change.

The fix: Ask a friend to be your accountability partner. This could look like sending a message to them after you've completed a pre-bed back mobility session, for example.

Behavioural patterns

People often have deeply ingrained behavioural patterns that are hard to break. These patterns can be the result of childhood experiences, past trauma or learned behaviours from family or cultural influences.

The fix: Have a think about your background and if there are any patterns or narratives you may have heard throughout this time. Write them down and use the tips in Chapter 4 to reframe the wording that you heard back then into how you might want to think about it now. See also the Useful Resources on page 275 if you need further support with this.

Not getting immediate pain relief

You may have tried some of the tips outlined in Part 2 but, after a few days, you haven't noticed a difference in your pain levels.

The fix: This is a big one I see with my clients, but your body takes time to adapt and become stronger. Please don't make changes for just one week and then assume they're not working. In a world where we are used to having access to food, taxis and our bank accounts in minutes, we have to remember to be patient with our bodies. Please don't give up, guys – it's all about consistency. (This is so important I've dedicated a whole section to it below.)

OSTEO TOP TIP

Grab a notebook or digital device and make a list under each of the above headings of what might be blocking you from doing the stuff you know your body needs. Quite often this exercise alone can be quite a revelation – just acknowledging that you have some barriers to change is a great motivator.

ISMAIL

Ismail had just graduated from university with first-class honours in Economics. He had landed an amazing job in London and came to see me with lower back pain and sciatic nerve pain down his right leg. He'd had this pain on and off for about six years, and it started when he was doing his GCSE exams.

I asked about his family's general health and well-being and he said that everyone in his immediate family was overweight, had diabetes, heart problems and arthritis.

I asked him what happened with his back pain when he was 16. He mentioned that his parents told him to ignore it and take painkillers, and they thought he was attention-seeking. They did eventually take him to the doctor, who wrote a letter requesting he be given extra time in his exams – so he could leave the exam hall to stretch – and gave him a referral to a physio. Ismail's parents said that physiotherapy didn't work and was a waste of time, and so Ismail found exercises on YouTube and did these himself at home to help relieve his symptoms.

The Ismail now sitting in front of me was overweight and deflated. He'd had the enthusiasm to implement more healthy behaviours into his life, but said he would start and then stop. He still lived at home and was consequently pulled back into the deeply ingrained belief that if he complained of pain he would be told he was attention-seeking and would also be discouraged from going to the gym.

I discussed this with Ismail and explained that his family's attitude might be limiting his ability to help his back in the long term. We decided together that he could call his friend who lived ten minutes away and join his gym to work out with him each week and try his best to avoid the conversations at home.

Ismail managed to lose almost 13kg in six months and enjoy a lifestyle that meant his back pain was drastically reduced – all from making one change: being accountable to someone who had the same interest in looking after their body.

The great thing is that Ismail's weight loss inspired his parents also to join a gym and start exercising more.

The Importance of Consistency

I've said it before and I'll say it again: healing your back pain is all about consistency. I know that it's often hard to do stuff when we can't see an immediate benefit – this is a very human reality. In our modern-day lives, we're always after the next quick fix, but the body is a well-tuned machine that responds to change gradually but surely, and so we need to be patient when we want it to recalibrate. Patience is a tough call these days when we live in a world of instant gratification. However, when it comes to healing your back, it's so important to give your body the time it requires to heal because everyone is different and it will be worth it in the long term (as frustrating as that can sometimes be).

When it comes to personal growth, whether that's incorporating mindfulness every day or doing your strengthening exercises, being consistent is the key to it all.

We all want results yesterday, but when it comes to preventative work on back pain, perseverance and consistency are key.

When you are in lots of pain, I know it can feel overwhelming, but taking gradual steps will help you to get back to doing what you love, and reduce your back pain. For example, setting an alarm to stand up and walk when you're working, writing in a journal for five minutes before bed, switching off your phone before you go to sleep or adding some turmeric to your food are all small steps that can take you towards your goals.

These small steps can be introduced gradually over time to

make a big difference in the long term. I'd encourage you to reflect on what you feel is manageable for you, your lifestyle and your level of back pain.

Managing a Flare-Up

Sometimes, despite all your hard work and following the principles outlined in the four steps, your pain flares up. If this happens, please know that it is quite common and is generally not a cause for alarm.

If you have a flare-up and you know that you are someone who panics and worries about your back pain, start by asking yourself the following questions:

1. In what way am I overestimating my ability to cope with this?
2. In what way am I underestimating my ability to cope with this?

These questions are amazing and I use them *a lot* in many things in my life. Basically, any time I panic or worry about stuff, I try to stop and ask myself these two questions.

What you realise very quickly is that you might remember a time when you've had a flare-up of back pain before. That actually it was awful then, but you got through it and you got moving and sleeping and working again.

In fact, you might think of a few times throughout your life when you have had injuries, surgery or severe pain. Your body pulled through every single time – even if it was rough!

When you ask yourself the second question about underestimating your ability to cope with it, you will realise that actually you coped every time. Ask yourself what would you do in the worst-case scenario? There is always a way out.

The reason I'm asking you to do this exercise is so that you don't panic if your pain flares up. You are more than capable of dealing with this.

Practical ways to deal with a flare-up

The sudden sharp pain

(The one where you bend over in the morning to put on your socks, you feel a sharp, knife-like pain and you are stuck and can't move without excruciating agony.)

- Try not to panic. Talk to yourself and remind yourself that it's OK; you are fine and your body is just adjusting to something.
- If you can't move the area at all – for example, you are stuck in a bent-over position or your neck is stuck straight without being able to turn left or right – try to reach some painkillers like ibuprofen. If you don't have those to hand, find a hot water bottle and put some heat on the area.
- Find a comfortable position, even if that is sitting on the side of a chair with your arm stuck above your head.
- After about 10–20 minutes, try to move slightly. Now it's probably going to hurt, but even moving a millimetre is better than nothing. The aim here is to remind your brain that it doesn't need to panic and that you still have movement and muscle strength.
- Keep moving as and when you can. I'm not asking you to really push yourself, but lean in to your pain slightly.

From my experience in clinic, I'd say that sharp pains tend to resolve themselves within a few days.

The gradual increase in pain that becomes unbearable

(The one where you feel invincible and convince yourself that you're all good, but then suddenly realise you can't now find a comfortable position to sleep or work or eat in. This is often referred to as 'creeper pain' as it can gradually creep up on you over the course of weeks, months or even years.)

- Try not to panic or get annoyed. You are not alone with creeper pain.
- Don't delay any further: Get some professional help from a doctor, osteopath, physiotherapist or chiropractor.
- Focus on what parts of your life are being impacted by this pain. If your sleep is being impacted, this is likely going to make you more irritable and feel more pain as a result, so first focus on how to get your sleep back (see Chapter 6 for advice on this).
- Try to focus on the positives and do not feel defeated by creeper pain. Do not let the pain win!

ETTA

Etta came to see me with creeper pain. She had had multiple episodes of pain that had crept up on her over the last 15 years.

This episode of pain was particularly bad. She had gone to a wedding four months previously and fallen on the dance floor. Having had a few wines, she didn't feel

---

anything at the time and just got up and carried on dancing, laughing it off.

Since then, the pain had gradually got worse, week on week. She had stopped wearing heels at weekends and going to her yoga class for the fear of making the pain worse. Now it was affecting her ability to sleep and she was finding it tough to find a comfortable position to sleep in.

I worked with her to help her understand that this pain probably stemmed from a long time ago. As we explored in Chapter 4, occasionally when you have a fall it can trigger the pain response in your body and this worry can keep it around for longer. Sometimes seeing a professional sooner is a great way of understanding what is going on and also getting reassurance on what movements you can do. This can give you some confidence to carry on doing the things that you love.

I told Etta to go back to yoga and that I would message her yoga teacher to explain her diagnosis so she could adapt the class for her. She was back in yoga within four days and, within a week, her back pain had gone.

I'm pleased to say that Etta hasn't had any more episodes in the last three years.

It's never too late to take steps to help heal your back.

Final Note

THIS BOOK HAS drawn on my years of experience helping those who are feeling lost and fearful about their back and spine. Back pain is an ever-increasing problem and it affects a staggering number of people worldwide. It's like the uninvited guest at a party, always showing up at the most inconvenient times and refusing to leave. Seriously, who invited this guy?

But, jokes aside, I know that back pain is no laughing matter. I'm hoping the information and quick tricks in this book have shown you how you can help yourself, even when you may not have much time. It's not easy to juggle pain, kids, work and a social life – I know.

In this day and age, where back pain seems to be more common than celebrity Instagram posts, it's important to talk about it. Share your experiences, seek advice and don't suffer in silence. There's strength in numbers, and we can kick back pain to the kerb. You have already taken your first steps towards healing your back pain by reading this book and implementing some of the tips in each chapter. Keep going! Small steps and commitment are going to lead to great, long-term results.

With a little movement, quality sleep, nutritious meals and a positive mindset, we can bid farewell to that uninvited guest and welcome a life of comfort and vitality. Here's to a pain-free back, and I wish you well on your journey ahead.

Useful Resources

Exercise Support

The NHS Couch to 5K app can help you get running: https://www.nhs.uk/live-well/exercise/running-and-aerobic-exercises/get-running-with-couch-to-5k/

The NHS website also has lots of general information about exercise: https://www.nhs.uk/live-well/exercise/

Mental Health Support

For immediate mental health support without talking, you can text SHOUT to 85258. Shout provides a confidential 24/7 text service for crisis support.

To discuss any upsetting issues, contact Samaritans at 116 123 (free from any phone), email jo@samaritans.org or visit their branches in person 24/7. The Samaritans Welsh Language Line is available at 0808 164 0123 from 7pm to 11pm daily.

For assistance with mental health issues, call SANEline at 0300 304 7000 between 4.30pm and 10.30pm daily, whether you're personally affected or supporting someone else.

There are also some excellent charities and organisations that you can reach out to if you need further support:

Mental Health Foundation: https://www.mentalhealth.org.uk/

Mental Health Mates: https://www.mentalhealthmates.co.uk/

Mind: https://www.mind.org.uk/

NHS Every Mind Matters: https://www.nhs.uk/every-mind-matters/

Nutrition Support

British Nutrition Foundation: https://www.nutrition.org.uk/

The Food Foundation: https://foodfoundation.org.uk

Osteopathy Support

If you'd like to hear more of my tips and general advice around all things osteopathy, please follow me on Instagram @osteoanisha.

If you'd like to book an appointment with me or a member of my team, go to: https://osteoanisha.com/

Alternatively, you can search the register for a local practitioner on the General Osteopathic Council's website: https://www.osteopathy.org.uk/home/

Pain Support

Backcare: https://backcare.org.uk/

The British Pain Society: https://www.britishpainsociety.org/

Healthtalk: https://healthtalk.org/

Pain Reprocessing Therapy: https://www.painreprocessing therapy.com

Pain UK: https://painuk.org/

Sleep Support

NHS: https://www.nhs.uk/every-mind-matters/mental-health-issues/sleep/

The Sleep Charity has a national sleep helpline: 03303 530 541. Their website also contains lots of useful information and support: https://thesleepcharity.org.uk/national-sleep-helpline/

Endnotes

Introduction

1 Walker BF. The prevalence of low back pain: a systematic review of the literature from 1966 to 1998. *J Spinal Disord*. 2000 Jun;13(3):205–17. doi: 10.1097/00002517-200006000-00003. PMID: 10872758.

2 https://www.unison.org.uk/get-help/knowledge/health-and-safety/back-pain

Chapter 1: How the Back Works

1 Bailey CA, Brooke-Wavell K. Optimum frequency of exercise for bone health: randomised controlled trial of a high-impact unilateral inter vention. *Bone*. 2010 Apr;46(4):1043–9. doi: 10.1016/j.bone.2009.12. 001. Epub 2010 Jan 6. PMID: 20004758.

2 Deyo RA, Weinstein JN. Low back pain. *N Engl J Med*. 2001;344: 363–70.

3 Deyo RA, Rainville J, Kent DL. What can the history and physical examination tell us about low back pain? *JAMA*. 1992;268:760–5.

4 Hart LG, Deyo RA, Cherkin DC. Physician office visits for low back pain. Frequency, clinical evaluation, and treatment patterns from a U.S. national survey. *Spine*. 1995;20:11–19.

5 Brinjikji W, et al. Systematic literature review of imaging features of spinal degeneration in asymptomatic populations. *AJNR Am J Neuroradiol*. 2015;36(4):811816. doi:10.3174/ajnr.A4173.

6 Kjaer P, Tunset A, Boyle E, Jensen TS. Progression of lumbar disc herniations over an eight-year period in a group of adult Danes from the general population: a longitudinal MRI study using quantitative measures. *BMC Musculoskelet Disord*. 2016 Jan 15;17(1):26.

7   Grundy PF, Roberts CJ. Does unequal leg length cause back pain? A case-control study. *Lancet.* 1984 Aug 4;2(8397):256–8.
8   Grob D, Frauenfelder H, Mannion AF. The association between cervical spine curvature and neck pain. *Eur Spine J.* 2007;16(5):669–78.

Chapter 2: Types of Back Pain

1   IASP-pain.org [Internet]. International Association for the Study of Pain. IASP Taxonomy; 2012 May 22.
2   Cohen SP, Mao J. Neuropathic pain: mechanisms and their clinical implications. *BMJ.* 2014;348:f7656.
3   Hashmi JA, et al. Shape shifting pain: chronification of back pain shifts brain representation from nociceptive to emotional circuits. *Brain.* 2013;136:2751–68.
4   Hulbert JC, et al. Inducing amnesia through systemic suppression. *Nat Commun.* 2015;7:1103. doi: 10.1038ncomms1103.
5   Australian Acute Musculoskeletal Pain Guidelines Group. Evidence-based management of acute musculoskeletal pain. Accessed 10 January 2007, at: http://www.nhmrc.gov.au/publications/_files/cp94.pdf.
6   Institute for Clinical Systems Improvement. Health care guideline: adult low back pain. 12th ed. September 2006. Accessed 10 January 2007.
7   van Tulder M, et al.; COST B13 Working Group on Guidelines for the Management of Acute Low Back Pain in Primary Care. Chapter 3. European guidelines for the management of acute nonspecific low back pain in primary care. *Eur Spine J.* 2006;15(suppl 2):S169–91.
8   Jarvik JG, Deyo RA. Diagnostic evaluation of low back pain with emphasis on imaging. *Ann Intern Med.* 2002;137:586–97.
9   Lirette LS, Chaiban G, Tolba R, Eissa H. Coccydynia: an overview of the anatomy, etiology, and treatment of coccyx pain. *Ochsner J.* 2014 Spring; 14(1):84–7. PMID: 24688338; PMCID: PMC3963058.
10 https://www.who.int/news-room/fact-sheets/detail/low-back-pain
11 Eck JC. Radiculopathy. Retrieved 12 April 2012.
12 Iversen T, et al. Accuracy of physical examination for chronic lumbar radiculopathy. *BMC Musculoskelet Disord.* 2013 Dec;14(1):1–9.
13 Hazlett JW. Low back pain with femoral neuritis. *Clin Orthop Relat Res.* 1975 May;(108):19–26. doi: 10.1097/00003086-197505000-00005. PMID: 124641.
14 Cho SC, Ferrante MA, Levin KH, Harmon RL, So YT. Utility of electrodiagnostic testing in evaluating patients with lumbosacral

radiculopathy: an evidence-based review. *Muscle Nerve.* 2010 Aug;42(2): 276–82.

15 Bogduk N. On the definitions and physiology of back pain, referred pain, and radicular pain. *Pain.* 2009;147(1):17–19.

16 Daley A. The role of exercise in the treatment of menstrual disorders: the evidence. *Br J Gen Pract.* 2009 Apr;59(561):241–2. doi: 10.3399/bjgp09X420301. PMID: 19341553; PMCID: PMC2662100.

17 https://www.ninds.nih.gov/health-information/disorders/back-pain

18 Green BN, Johnson CD, Snodgrass J, Smith M, Dunn AS. Association between smoking and back pain in a cross-section of adult Americans. *Cureus.* 2016 Sep 26;8(9):e806. doi: 10.7759/cureus.806. PMID: 27790393; PMCID: PMC5081254.

19 Eck JC. 2012.

20 Cho SC. 2010.

21 Leininger B, Bronfort G, Evans R, Reiter T. Spinal manipulation or mobilization for radiculopathy: a systematic review. *Phys Med Rehabil Clin N Am.* 2011 Feb 1;22(1):105–25.

22 Young IA, Pozzi F, Dunning J, Linkonis R, Michener LA. Immediate and short-term effects of thoracic spine manipulation in patients with cervical radiculopathy: a randomized controlled trial. *JOSPT.* 2019 May;49(5): 299–309.

23 Bogduk N. 2009.

24 https://www.who.int/news-room/fact-sheets/detail/low-back-pain

25 Andersson GB. The epidemiology of spinal disorders. In: *The Adult Spine: Principles and Practice.* Frymoyer JW (ed.) (Philadelphia, 1997).

26 Cherkin DC, Deyo RA, Street JH, Barlow W. Predicting poor outcomes for back pain seen in primary care using patients' own criteria. *Spine.* 1996 Dec 15;21(24):2900–7.

27 Epping-Jordan JE, et al. Transition to chronic pain in men with low back pain: predictive relationships among pain intensity, disability, and depressive symptoms. *Health Psychol.* 1998 Sep;17(5):421.

28 Bair MJ, Robinson RL, Katon W, Kroenke K. Depression and pain comorbidity: a literature review. *Arch Intern Med.* 2003;163(20):2433–45.

29 Deyo RA, Bass JE. Lifestyle and low-back pain. The influence of smoking and obesity. *Spine.* 1989 May;14(5):501–6.

Chapter 3: Step 1: Keep Moving

1 https://www.nhs.uk/live-well/exercise/exercise-health-benefits/
2 Reiner M, et al. Long-term health benefits of physical activity – a

systematic review of longitudinal studies. *BMC Public Health.* 2013;13:813. https://doi.org/10.1186/1471-2458-13-813.

3   Kroll HR. Exercise therapy for chronic pain. *Phys Med Rehabil Clin N Am.* 2015 May;26(2):263–81. doi: 10.1016/j.pmr.2014.12.007. Epub 2015 Feb 21. PMID: 25952064.

4   Gordon R, Bloxham S. A systematic review of the effects of exercise and physical activity on non-specific chronic low back pain. *Healthcare (Basel).* 2016 Apr 25;4(2):22. doi: 10.3390/healthcare4020022. PMID: 27417610; PMCID: PMC4934575.

5   Muzin S, Isaac Z, Walker J, Abd OE, Baima J. When should a cervical collar be used to treat neck pain? *Curr Rev Musculoskelet Med.* 2008 Jun;1(2):114–19. doi: 10.1007/s12178-007-9017-9. PMID: 19468883; PMCID: PMC2684205.

6   Ibid.

7   Koes BW, van Tulder MW, Peul WC. Diagnosis and treatment of sciatica. *BMJ.* 2007 Jun 23;334(7607):1313–17. doi: 10.1136/bmj.39223.428495. BE. PMID: 17585160; PMCID: PMC1895638.

8   Simic L, Sarabon N, Markovic G. Does pre-exercise static stretching inhibit maximal muscular performance? A meta-analytical review. *Scand J Med Sci Sports.* 2013 Mar;23(2):131–48. doi: 10.1111/j.1600-0838.2012.01444.x. Epub 2012 Feb 8. PMID: 22316148.

9   Iwata M, et al. Dynamic stretching has sustained effects on range of motion and passive stiffness of the hamstring muscles. *J Sports Sci Med.* 2019 Feb 11;18(1):13–20. PMID: 30787647; PMCID: PMC6370952.

10   Andersen JC. Stretching before and after exercise: effect on muscle soreness and injury risk. *J Athl Train.* 2005 Jul–Sep;40(3):218–20. PMID: 16284645; PMCID: PMC1250267.

11   Tsutsumi T, Don BM, Zaichkowsky LD, Takenaka K, Oka K, Ohno T. Comparison of high and moderate intensity of strength training on mood and anxiety in older adults. Percept Mot Skills. 1998;87(3):1003–11. https://doi.org/10.2466/pms.1998.87.3.1003.

12   Green LA, Gabriel DA. The cross education of strength and skill following unilateral strength training in the upper and lower limbs. *J Neurophysiol.* 2018 Aug 1;120(2):468–79. doi: 10.1152/jn.00116.2018. Epub 2018 Apr 18. PMID: 29668382; PMCID: PMC6139459.

13   Ma J, et al. Effect of aquatic physical therapy on chronic low back pain: a systematic review and meta-analysis. *BMC Musculoskelet Disord.* 2022;23:1050.

14   Alentorn-Geli E, Samuelsson K, Musahl V, Green CL, Bhandari M, Karlsson J. The association of recreational and competitive running with

hip and knee osteoarthritis: a systematic review and meta-analysis. *J Orthop Sports Phys Ther*. 2017 Jun;47(6):373–90. doi: 10.2519/jospt. 2017.7137. Epub 2017 May 13. PMID: 28504066.

15 Bishop M, Fiolkowski P, Conrad B, Brunt D, Horodyski M. Athletic footwear, leg stiffness, and running kinematics. *J Athl Train*. 2006 Oct-Dec;41(4):387–92. PMID: 17273463; PMCID: PMC1748411.

Chapter 4: Step 2: Reset Your Mind

1 Chu B, et al. Physiology, Stress Reaction. [Updated 2022 Sep 12]. In: StatPearls [Internet]. Treasure Island (FL): StatPearls Publishing; 2024.

2 Hannibal KE, Bishop MD. Chronic stress, cortisol dysfunction, and pain: a psychoneuroendocrine rationale for stress management in pain rehabilitation. *Phys Ther*. 2014 Dec;94(12):1816–25. doi: 10.2522/ptj. 20130597. Epub 2014 Jul 17. PMID: 25035267; PMCID: PMC4263906.

3 Ibid.

4 Ibid.

5 Ibid.

6 Lumley MA, et al. Pain and emotion: a biopsychosocial review of recent research. *J Clin Psychol*. 2011 Sep;67(9):942–68. doi: 10.1002/ jclp.20816. Epub 2011 Jun 6. PMID: 21647882; PMCID: PMC 3152687.

7 Baird A, Sheffield D. The relationship between pain beliefs and physical and mental health outcome measures in chronic low back pain: direct and indirect effects. *Healthcare (Basel)*. 2016 Aug 19;4(3):58. doi: 10. 3390/healthcare4030058. PMID: 27548244; PMCID: PMC5041059.

8 Madison A, Kiecolt-Glaser JK. Stress, depression, diet, and the gut microbiota: human-bacteria interactions at the core of psycho neuroimmunology and nutrition. *Curr Opin Behav Sci*. 2019 Aug;28: 105–10. doi: 10.1016/j.cobeha.2019.01.011. Epub 2019 Mar 25. PMID: 32395568; PMCID: PMC7213601.

9 Keng SL, Smoski MJ, Robins CJ. Effects of mindfulness on psychological health: a review of empirical studies. *Clin Psychol Rev*. 2011 Aug;31(6): 1041–56. doi: 10.1016/j.cpr.2011.04.006. Epub 2011 May 13. PMID: 21802619; PMCID: PMC3679190.

10 Ozbay F, Johnson DC, Dimoulas E, Morgan CA, Charney D, Southwick S. Social support and resilience to stress: from neurobiology to clinical practice. *Psychiatry (Edgmont)*. 2007 May;4(5):35–40. PMID: 20806 028; PMCID: PMC2921311.

11 Lumley MA. 2011.

12 Conversano C, Rotondo A, Lensi E, Della Vista O, Arpone F, Reda MA. Optimism and its impact on mental and physical well-being. *Clin Pract Epidemiol Ment Health.* 2010 May 14;6:25–9. doi: 10.2174/17450 17901006010025. PMID: 20592964; PMCID: PMC2894461.

13 Franchignoni F, Giordano A, Ferriero G, Monticone M. Measurement precision of the Pain Catastrophizing Scale and its short forms in chronic low back pain. *Sci Rep.* 2022 Jul 14;12(1):12042. doi: 10.1038/s41598-022-15522-x. PMID: 35835830; PMCID: PMC9283330.

Chapter 5: Step 3: Eat Well

1 https://www.rehabmedicine.pitt.edu/sites/default/files/enrico.pdf

2 https://www.ncbi.nlm.nih.gov/pmc/articles/PMC3257651/

3 Cordingley DM, Cornish SM. Omega-3 fatty acids for the management of osteoarthritis: a narrative review. *Nutrients.* 2022 Aug 16;14(16):3362. doi: 10.3390/nu14163362. PMID: 36014868; PMCID: PMC9413343.

4 https://www.ncbi.nlm.nih.gov/pmc/articles/PMC3249911/

5 https://www.ncbi.nlm.nih.gov/pmc/articles/PMC5664031/

6 Lee JY, Zhao L, Hwang DH. Modulation of pattern recognition receptor-mediated inflammation and risk of chronic diseases by dietary fatty acids. *Nutr Rev.* 2010;68:38–61.

7 https://www.sciencedirect.com/science/article/pii/S2161831322009267#bib17

8 Calder PC. Omega-3 fatty acids and inflammatory processes. *Nutrients.* 2010 Mar;2(3):355–74. doi: 10.3390/nu2030355. Epub 2010 Mar 18. PMID: 22254027; PMCID: PMC3257651.

9 Innes JK, Calder PC. Omega-6 fatty acids and inflammation. *Prostaglandins Leukot Essent Fatty Acids.* 2018 May;132:41–8. doi: 10.1016/j.plefa.2018.03.004. Epub 2018 Mar 22. PMID: 29610056.

10 Song M, et al. A comparison of the burden of knee osteoarthritis attributable to high body mass index in China and globally from 1990 to 2019. *Front Med (Lausanne).* 2023 Aug 23;10:1200294. doi: 10.3389/fmed.2023.1200294. PMID: 37680622; PMCID: PMC 10481341.

11 https://www.nhs.uk/live-well/eat-well/food-guidelines-and-food-labels/the-eatwell-guide/

12 https://www.ncbi.nlm.nih.gov/pmc/articles/PMC9228511/

13 https://www.ncbi.nlm.nih.gov/pmc/articles/PMC8754590/

14 Essouiri J, Harzy T, Benaicha N, Errasfa M, Abourazzak FE. Effectiveness of argan oil consumption on knee osteoarthritis symptoms: a randomized

controlled clinical trial. *Curr Rheumatol Rev* 2017;13:231–5. doi: 10.21 74/1573397113666170710123031.

15 Bitler CM, et al. Olive extract supplement decreases pain and improves daily activities in adults with osteoarthritis and decreases plasma homocysteine in those with rheumatoid arthritis. *Nutr Res.* 2007;27: 470–7. doi: 10.1016/j.nutres.2007.06.003.

16 Berbert AA, Kondo CR, Almendra CL, Matsuo T, Dichi I. Supplementation of fish oil and olive oil in patients with rheumatoid arthritis. *Nutrition.* 2005;21:131–6. doi: 10.1016/j.nut.2004.03.023.

17 Hill CL, et al. Fish oil in knee osteoarthritis: a randomised clinical trial of low dose versus high dose. *Ann Rheum Dis.* 2016;75:23–9. doi: 10.1136/ annrheumdis-2014-207169.

18 Peanpadungrat P. Efficacy and safety of fish oil in treatment of knee osteoarthritis. *J Med Assoc Thai.* 2015;98(suppl 3):S110–14.

19 Gray P, Chappell A, Jenkinson AM, Thies F, Gray SR. Fish oil supplementation reduces markers of oxidative stress but not muscle soreness after eccentric exercise. *Int J Sport Nutr Exerc Metab.* 2014; 24:206–14. doi: 10.1123/ijsnem.2013-0081.

20 Tartibian B, Maleki BH, Abbasi A. The effects of ingestion of omega-3 fatty acids on perceived pain and external symptoms of delayed onset muscle soreness in untrained men. *Clin J Sport Med.* 2009;19:115–19. doi: 10.1097/JSM.0b013e31819b51b3.

21 Tsuchiya Y, Yanagimoto K, Nakazato K, Hayamizu K, Ochi E. Eicosapentaenoic and docosahexaenoic acids-rich fish oil supplementation attenuates strength loss and limited joint range of motion after eccentric contractions: a randomized, double-blind, placebo-controlled, parallel-group trial. *Eur J Appl Physiol.* 2016;116:1179–88. doi: 10.1007/ s00421-016-3373-3.

22 https://www.ncbi.nlm.nih.gov/pmc/articles/PMC5664031/

23 https://www.nhs.uk/live-well/eat-well/food-types/fish-and-shellfish-nutrition/

24 https://pubmed.ncbi.nlm.nih.gov/27676659/

25 https://www.nhs.uk/conditions/vitamins-and-minerals/vitamin-d/

26 https://www.ncbi.nlm.nih.gov/pmc/articles/PMC7400867/

27 Wax B, Kerksick CM, Jagim AR, Mayo JJ, Lyons BC, Kreider RB. Creatine for exercise and sports performance, with recovery considerations for healthy populations. *Nutrients.* 2021 Jun 2;13(6):1915. doi: 10.3390/ nu13061915. PMID: 34199588; PMCID: PMC8228369.

28 https://pubmed.ncbi.nlm.nih.gov/11735088/

29 Watanabe A, Kato N, Kato T. Effects of creatine on mental fatigue and cerebral hemoglobin oxygenation. *Neurosci Res.* 2002 Apr.

30 McMorris T, et al. Effect of creatine supplementation and sleep deprivation, with mild exercise, on cognitive and psychomotor performance, mood state, and plasma concentrations of catecholamines and cortisol. *Psychopharmacology (Berl).* 2006 Mar.

31 Cooper R, Naclerio F, Allgrove J, Jimenez A. Creatine supplementation with specific view to exercise/sports performance: an update. *J Int Soc Sports Nutr.* 2012 Jul 20;9(1):33. doi: 10.1186/1550-2783-9-33. PMID: 22817979; PMCID: PMC3407788.

32 https://pubmed.ncbi.nlm.nih.gov/30498758/

33 Belcaro G, et al. Efficacy and safety of Meriva(R), a curcumin-phosphatidylcholine complex, during extended administration in osteoarthritis patients. *Altern Med Rev.* 2010;15(4):337–44.

34 https://www.ncbi.nlm.nih.gov/pmc/articles/PMC5337510/

35 https://journals.lww.com/behaviouralpharm/Abstract/2019/04000/ Stress_and_the_gut_microbiota_brain_axis.9.aspx

36 https://www.ncbi.nlm.nih.gov/pmc/articles/PMC6511407/

37 Ibid.

38 https://www.sciencedirect.com/science/article/pii/S0092867415002482

39 https://www.sciencedirect.com/science/article/pii/S0007091219306385

40 Whorwell PJ, McCallum M, Creed FH, Roberts CT. Non-colonic features of irritable bowel syndrome. *Gut.* 1986 Jan;27(1):37–40. doi: 10.1136/gut.27.1.37. PMID: 3949235; PMCID: PMC1433171.

41 https://www.ncbi.nlm.nih.gov/pmc/articles/PMC6139698/

42 Steer S, et al. Low back pain, sacroiliitis, and the relationship with HLA-B27 in Crohn's disease. *J Rheumatol.* 2003 Mar;30(3):518–22.

43 Sophia Fox AJ, Bedi A, Rodeo SA. The basic science of articular cartilage: structure, composition, and function. *Sports Health.* 2009 Nov;1(6): 461–8. doi: 10.1177/1941738109350438. PMID: 23015907; PMCID: PMC3445147.

44 https://journals.lww.com/anesthesia-analgesia/FullText/2014/06000/De hydration_Enhances_Pain_Evoked_Activation_in_the.23.aspx

45 https://onlinelibrary.wiley.com/doi/10.1111/psyp.12610

Chapter 6: Step 4: Sleep Better

1 Stepan ME, Altmann EM, Fenn KM. Effects of total sleep deprivation on procedural placekeeping: more than just lapses of attention. *J Exp Psychol Gen.* 2020;149(4):800–6.

2 https://www.nuffieldhealth.com/healthiernation

3 Nutt D, Wilson S, Paterson L. Sleep disorders as core symptoms of depression. *Dialogues Clin Neurosci*. 2008;10(3):329–36.

4 Mathias JL, Cant ML, Burke A. Sleep disturbances and sleep disorders in adults living with chronic pain: a meta-analysis. *Sleep Med*. 2018; 52:198–210. https://doi.org/10.1016/j.sleep.2018.05.023

5 https://pubmed.ncbi.nlm.nih.gov/31149975/; https://pubmed.ncbi.nlm.nih.gov/28940629/

6 https://pubmed.ncbi.nlm.nih.gov/22547894/

7 Gerhart et al. Relationships Between Sleep Quality and Pain-Related Factors for People with Chronic Low Back Pain: Tests of Reciprocal and Time of Day Effects, www.ncbi.nlm.nih.gov/pmc/articles/PMC5846493/.

8 Srinivasan V, Zakaria R, Jeet Singh H, Acuna-Castroviejo D. Melatonin and its agonists in pain modulation and its clinical application. *Arch Ital Biol*. 2012 Dec;150(4):274–89. doi: 10.4449/aib.v150i4.1391. PMID: 23479460.

9 https://www.ncbi.nlm.nih.gov/pmc/articles/PMC3548567/

10 https://www.ncbi.nlm.nih.gov/pmc/articles/PMC9289983/

11 Finan PH, Goodin BR, Smith MT. The association of sleep and pain: an update and a path forward. *J Pain*. 2013 Dec;14(12):1539–52. doi: 10.1016/j.jpain.2013.08.007. PMID: 24290442; PMCID: PMC4046588.

12 Gordon S, Grimmer K, Trott P. Sleep position, age, gender, sleep quality and waking cervico-thoracic symptoms. *Internet J Allied Health Sci Pract*. 2007;5.

13 Woo AK. Depression and anxiety in pain. *Rev Pain*. 2010 Mar;4(1): 8–12. doi: 10.1177/204946371000400103. PMID: 26527193; PMCID: PMC4590059.

14 Somers TJ, et al. Pain catastrophizing and pain-related fear in osteoarthritis patients: relationships to pain and disability. *J Pain Symptom Manage*. 2009 May;37(5):863–72. doi: 10.1016/j.jpainsymman.2008.05.009. Epub 2008 Nov 28. PMID: 19041218; PMCID: PMC2702756.

15 Alhalal EA, Alhalal IA, Alaida AM, Alhweity SM, Alshojaa AY, Alfaori AT. Effects of chronic pain on sleep quality and depression: A cross-sectional study. *Saudi Med J*. 2021 Mar;42(3):315–323. doi: 10.15537/smj.42.3.20200768. PMID: 33632911; PMCID: PMC7989257.

16 Chand SP, Kuckel DP, Huecker MR. Cognitive Behavior Therapy. [Updated 2023 May 23]. In: StatPearls [Internet]. Treasure Island (FL): StatPearls Publishing; 2023.

17 https://www.ncbi.nlm.nih.gov/pmc/articles/PMC3181635/

18   Irish LA, Kline CE, Gunn HE, Buysse DJ, Hall MH. The role of sleep hygiene in promoting public health: a review of empirical evidence. *Sleep Med Rev.* 2015;22:23–36.

19   Steffens D, et al. What triggers an episode of acute low back pain? A case-crossover study. *Arthritis Care Res (Hoboken).* 2015 Mar;67(3): 403–10. PMID: 25665074.

20   Gohil BC, Rosenblum LA, Coplan JD, Kral JG. Hypothalamic-pituitary-adrenal axis function and the metabolic syndrome X of obesity. *CNS Spectr.* 2001 Jul;6(7):581–6, 589. PMID: 15573024.

21   Franceschi C, Campisi J. Chronic inflammation (inflammaging) and its potential contribution to age-associated diseases. *J Gerontol A Biol Sci Med Sci.* 2014 Jun;69(suppl 1):S4–9. PMID: 24833586; PainSci Bibliography: 53291.

22   https://www.gov.uk/government/news/new-review-launched-into-vitamin-d-intake-to-help-tackle-health-disparities

23   Holick MF, Chen TC. Vitamin D deficiency: a worldwide problem with health consequences. *Am J Clin Nutr.* 2008 Apr;87(4):1080S–6S. PMID: 18400738; PainSci Bibliography: 55028.

Chapter 7: Treatment Options

1   Kumar S, Beaton K, Hughes T. The effectiveness of massage therapy for the treatment of nonspecific low back pain: a systematic review. *Int J Gen Med.* 2013 Sep 4;6:733–41. doi: 10.2147/IJGM.S50243. PMID: 24043951; PMCID: PMC3772691.

2   Deflorin C, Hohenauer E, Stoop R, van Daele U, Clijsen R, Taeymans J. Physical management of scar tissue: a systematic review and meta-analysis. *J Altern Complement Med.* 2020 Oct;26(10):854–65. doi: 10.1089/acm.2020.0109. Epub 2020 Jun 24. PMID: 32589450; PMCID: PMC7578190.

3   Vickers AJ, et al. Acupuncture for chronic pain: individual patient data meta-analysis. *Arch Intern Med.* 2012;172(19):1444–53. doi:10.1001/archinternmed.2012.3654.

4   Yin J, Yuan Q, Xiang Z. Effects of transcutaneous electrical nerve stimulation on patients with chronic low back pain: a systematic review and meta-analysis of randomized controlled trials. *Disabil Rehabil.* 2019;41(5):574–85. doi: 10.1080/09638288.2017.1410730.

5   Shiri R, Coggon D, Falah-Hassani K. Exercise for the prevention of low back pain: systematic review and meta-analysis of controlled trials. *Am J Epidemiol.* 2018 May;187(5):1093–110.

6 Bronfort G, et al. Effectiveness of manual therapies: the UK evidence report. *Chiropr Man Therap.* 2010;18:3.

7 O'Hagan ET, Cashin AG, Traeger AC, McAuley JH. Person-centred education and advice for people with low back pain: making the best of what we know. *Braz J Phys Ther.* 2023 Jan–Feb;27(1):100478. doi: 10.1016/j.bjpt.2022.100478. Epub 2022 Dec 22. PMID: 36657216; PMCID: PMC9868342.

8 Kurebayashi LF, Turrini RN, Souza TP, Takiguchi RS, Kuba G, Nagumo MT. Massage and reiki used to reduce stress and anxiety: randomized clinical trial. *Rev Lat Am Enfermagem.* 2016 Nov 28;24:e2834. doi: 10.1590/1518-8345.1614.2834. PMID: 27901219; PMCID: PMC5172615.

9 Kamioka H, et al. Effectiveness of aquatic exercise and balneotherapy: a summary of systematic reviews based on randomized controlled trials of water immersion therapies. *J Epidemiol.* 2010:20(1):2–12.

10 Knechtle B, Waśkiewicz Z, Sousa CV, Hill L, Nikolaidis PT. Cold water swimming-benefits and risks: a narrative review. *Int J Environ Res Public Health.* 2020 Dec 2;17(23):8984. doi: 10.3390/ijerph17238984. PMID: 33276648; PMCID: PMC7730683.

11 Lateef F. Post exercise ice water immersion: is it a form of active recovery? *J Emerg Trauma Shock.* 2010 Jul;3(3):302. doi: 10.4103/0974-2700.665 70. PMID: 20930987; PMCID: PMC2938508.

12 Thompson et al. The effectiveness of hypnosis for pain relief: a systematic review and meta-analysis of 85 controlled experimental trials. *Neurosci Biobehav Rev.* 2019;99.

13 Eskander JP, Spall J, Spall A, Shah RV, Kaye AD. Cannabidiol (CBD) as a treatment of acute and chronic back pain: a case series and literature review. *J Opioid Manag.* 2020 May/Jun;16(3):215–18. doi: 10.5055/jom.2020.0570. PMID: 32421842.

14 Haltner-Ukomadu E, Sacha M, Richter A, Hussein K. Hydrogel increases diclofenac skin permeation and absorption. *Biopharm Drug Dispos.* 2019 Jul;40(7):217–24. doi: 10.1002/bdd.2194. Epub 2019 Jul 18. PMID: 31242332; PMCID: PMC6771745.

15 Eskander JP. 2020.

16 Hall AM, Aubrey-Bassler K, Thorne B, Maher CG. Do not routinely offer imaging for uncomplicated low back pain. *BMJ.* 2021 Feb 12; 372:n291. doi: 10.1136/bmj.n291. PMID: 33579691; PMCID: PMC80 23332.

17 Ibid.

18 Brinjikji W, et al. MRI findings of disc degeneration are more prevalent in adults with low back pain than in asymptomatic controls: a systematic

review and meta-analysis. *AJNR Am J Neuroradiol.* 2015 Dec;36(12): 2394–9. doi: 10.3174/ajnr.A4498. Epub 2015 Sep 10. PMID: 26359154; PMCID: PMC7964277.

19 Keuss SE, et al. Incidental findings on brain imaging and blood tests: results from the first phase of Insight 46, a prospective observational substudy of the 1946 British birth cohort. *BMJ Open.* 2019;9:e029502. doi:10.1136/ bmjopen-2019-029502.

20 Wallace MK, Jeanblanc AB, Musil CM. Incidental findings: a practical protocol for reporting elevated depressive symptoms in behavioral health research. *Arch Psychiatr Nurs.* 2020 Jun;34(3):96–9. doi: 10.1016/j. apnu.2020.04.005. Epub 2020 Apr 13. PMID: 32513473; PMCID: PMC7323861.

21 Wang ZR, Ni GX. Is it time to put traditional cold therapy in rehabilitation of soft-tissue injuries out to pasture? *World J Clin Cases.* 2021 Jun 16;9(17):4116–22. doi: 10.12998/wjcc.v9.i17.4116. PMID: 34141774; PMCID: PMC8173427.

22 Dubois B, Esculier J. Soft-tissue injuries simply need PEACE and LOVE. *Br J Sports Med.* 2020;54:72–3. https://bjsm.bmj.com/content/54/2/72. abstract

23 Moghaddami M, Kamyab M, Rezasoltani A. The effect of heat therapy on low back pain: A systematic review and meta-analysis. *Clin Rehabil.* 2019;33(4):589–99. doi: 10.1177/0269215519826052.

Acknowledgements

In 2019, I decided to write a list of dreams that I wanted to achieve and on that list was 'Be a published author'. It seems fitting to thank the whiteboard I used to look at every day with this list on, as it really is a dream come true, writing this book.

This journey, the creation of this book, has been a joy and, at the same time, one of the hardest things I have ever done. I could not have done it alone and so I want to express my deepest gratitude to those who have stood by my side, providing support and inspiration at every step of the way.

First and foremost, I want to thank my parents, who have been the pillars of my life. Their unwavering support and belief in me have been my driving force. I am endlessly grateful for the love and encouragement they have given me, writing this book and in life.

To my big sister, Reena, you are my eternal inspiration. Your determination, unconditional love and osteopathic support have not only enriched my life, but also fuelled my passion for this project. Your way of being in this world is a constant reminder of what's possible.

To the team of talented therapists and staff who have helped to cover for me, support me and continue to provide such a high level of care to our patients across our clinics.

To my extended family and friends, you have shared

countless meals, phone calls and messages with me during this journey. Your support and patience as I tried to juggle a business, my patients and the writing of this book mean more to me than words can express.

Elly James, my agent, saw something in me and pushed me to believe I could write a book. Your belief in my abilities gave me the confidence to forge ahead.

To Sam Jackson and Anya Hayes at Vermilion, your patience and positive reinforcement helped to keep me focused and believe in my ability to write this book.

To my editor Julia Kellaway, who put up with me on numerous calls, who built me up when I felt scared and whose hard work has been instrumental in bringing this book to life.

I am grateful for the opportunity to work with such a dedicated team and couldn't have done it without you.

To my clients, who have always supported and believed in me, you've made me feel like I can do anything. This book is a testament to the trust you've placed in me over the years, and these pages really are inspired by you.

About the Author

Award-winning Anisha Joshi graduated as an osteopath 14 years ago and quickly realised she was passionate about educating people about their bodies. She has since been on a mission to rid the world of its aching spine and at the age of 24 opened a clinic, which she tripled in size in just five years. She now owns four clinics treating more than 1,000 patients a year with her osteopath sister and highly skilled team of practitioners in Central London, Hertfordshire, Berkshire and Surrey.

Anisha has a unique approach to wellness as she looks at the body as a whole. With research now showing that things like sleep and stress have an impact on how people experience pain, Anisha has found that implementing this within her clinic and on her social media platforms has enabled her to make a bigger impact on people's lives.

Anisha wants to make bone and back health more relatable and help people to recognise that pain is not to be feared and is as common as getting a cold. Our bodies are strong, but they just get sore sometimes, and Anisha's mission is to reduce the fear associated with pain and help people help themselves at home, while adding a bit of humour into the mix.

Index